Schools and the Health of Children

Dedicated to the memory of Marcia Lynn Whicker, my friend and colleague with whom I wrote many books, analyzed many colleagues, and shared many special times (both good and bad). You are missed.

Jennie Jacobs Kronenfeld

Schools and the Health of Children

Protecting Our Future

Sage Publications, Inc.
International Educational and Professional Publisher
Thousand Oaks ▪ London ▪ New Delhi

For information:

Sage Publications, Inc.
2455 Teller Road
Thousand Oaks, California 91320
E-mail: order@sagepub.com

Sage Publications Ltd.
6 Bonhill Street
London EC2A 4PU
United Kingdom

Sage Publications India Pvt. Ltd.
M-32 Market
Greater Kailash I
New Delhi 110 048 India

Printed in the United States of America

Library of Congress Cataloging-in-Publication Data

Kronenfeld, Jennie J.
    Schools and the health of children: Protecting our future / by Jennie Jacobs Kronenfeld.
        p. cm.
    Includes bibliographical references and index.
    ISBN 0-7619-1113-8 (cloth: alk. paper)
    ISBN 0-7619-1114-6 (pbk.: alk. paper)
        1. School health services—United States. 2. School children—Health and hygiene—United States. 3. Health education—United States. I. Title.
    LB3409.U5 K76 1999
    371.7'1'0973—dc21   99-6313

00 01 02 03 04 05 06 7 6 5 4 3 2 1

Acquiring Editor:	Peter Labella
Editorial Assistant:	Renée Piernot
Production Editor:	Diana E. Axelsen
Editorial Assistant:	Patricia Zeman

TABLE OF CONTENTS

LIST OF TABLES

PREFACE

Children occupy unique positions in modern American society. On one hand, we idealize children and childhood, viewing it as the most innocent and carefree time of life, a time free from everyday worries about the necessities of life. However, this is not the reality of childhood for a substantial number of American children. Almost one quarter of US children live in poverty, and children are the age group in American society most likely to live in poverty. Also, children under the age of 18 account for most of the loss of dependents being covered through health insurance plans at the workplace. Thus, the topic of this book, the health of children and school health programs, are an important issue in American society.

In many ways, schools are an underused resource in the lives of children. At a time when two-parent families generally have both adults working most of the day, and the majority of children will spend part of their childhood in a single-parent home, many schools have not acknowledged this change in the lives at home of most children. Most children in the US from ages 5-18 now spend a major part of their days in schools, but many localities still have a limited view of what schools can provide for children. Obviously, they are to provide education. Federally funded food programs have created a societal agreement that schools should provide an opportunity to buy lunch for all children, and the provision of free lunches and breakfast for many poor children. Increasingly, some elementary schools are providing extended care for younger children, to deal with the issue of "latchkey" children who have no adult at home when the child returns from a typical school day. Many schools, however, do not view their roles as dealing with the "whole" child, including whether they have food to eat at home, school supplies, clothing, an adult to help them in the afternoon, and medical care if they need it. This statement is not meant to castigate schools, or caring individual teachers or principals. In fact, we all know that many schools are filled with caring teachers who give lunch money to a child who forgets it, buy supplies for children who seem to have less than others, and bring in gently used clothing and toys from their own children to distribute to certain children in their classes.

In my own experience as a parent of school-aged children, first in South Carolina and now in Arizona, I have talked to principals who told me about the extra parts of their job. Often, the principal at the end of the day ended up delivering children home because a parent never showed to pick the child up. Sometimes principals allowed a child to stay and work in the library at school until all staff left because they knew the child was fearful of going home to a cold, empty apartment until closer to the time the parent arrived from work.

These examples of caring, individual teachers and principals can be found across the nation. They are examples of the best models of caring and concern in American society. As a formal system, however, schools often are only able to deal with limited needs of children. Health care in a school setting has ranged from as little as the placement of bandaids and taking of temperatures to better trained nurses who have tried to advocate for the children in their school and call doctors' offices to try and help children obtain health care.

This book is about expanded models for schools in the lives of children, especially focused on the health care needs of children. As part of a local foundation's goal to help provide health care services for more children in Arizona, I became the evaluator of a project of school-based health clinics in the state of Arizona. These were not the first of such clinics in the nation, nor even the very first in Arizona (although there were only a few fledgling examples before the project was begun that is described in detail in Chapter 5 of this book). As I worked with these projects and helped them to develop data systems to collect information, as well as conducted interviews with school nursing and educational personnel, I realized that my previous experience in health prevention projects and projects with child injury had provided important background for this project. My research on issues of access to care and health insurance was also important, because one of the advantages of school based clinics for many children and their families is the immediate availability of help and the ability of school nurses to help serve as advocates for the interest of their children.

For some parents, the health care system is a complicated place, one difficult to access not only due to lack of money and transportation, but due to language limitations and lack of knowledge of health care. Parents have to learn to use the school system (it is required by law that children attend, generally to age 16, and most parents view schools as very important for the chances of children to have a better life as adults). Although some areas have busing to schools, most children in the nation attend elementary schools near their homes and in places where the staff develop some understanding of the needs to their area. This book presents examples of how school-based clinics have worked in one state with several different types of models. These models are presented after a review of child health and school health programs. As a new program to help provide health insurance to some of the working poor (Child Health Insurance Program - [CHIP]) began in many states in 1999, a book that examines the health of children and roles that schools can play in improving the health of children addressed a topic that is especially timely. The topic is also, in some ways, timeless, because the health of children should also be of special concern in a caring society. Children represent the future of any country, and access to health care provides children with an opportunity for a decent start in life.

ACKNOWLEDGMENTS

I would like to acknowledge the assistance of several groups and people who helped to make this book possible. Without the grant from the Flinn Foundation, I would not have become so involved in the issue of school-based health services. I wish to thank the Flinn Foundation both for helping to stimulate my interest and for providing the funds for the many site visits that I conducted to each of the projects. Special thanks within the Flinn Foundation goes to Myra Millinger, the program officer with whom I worked most closely. She always helped with thoughtful comments while the grant was underway, and she is most knowledgeable about issues of school health and adolescent health in the state of Arizona.

I would also like to thank my university, Arizona State University, Larry Penley, dean of my College of Business, and Eugene Schneller, the chairperson of my unit, the School of Health Administration and Policy, during the years I was most involved in writing this book, for helping to facilitate the sabbatical that made the completion of the book possible. For detailed support, I am most appreciative to Matthew Brown, my graduate assistant, who was always willing to try and hunt down more references and statistics, whether in the library or over internet.

I would also like to thank my family for their patience, as I often stated that I needed to go write and not be bothered with other details. My husband, Michael Kronenfeld, has always been supportive and has read outlines of the proposed book and versions of several of the chapters. My sons, Shaun, Jeffrey, and Aaron, though less patient, generally did respect my need for my materials to be left alone (aided during this project by the addition of computers in their bedrooms).

CHAPTER 1

INTRODUCTION

The health of children is one of those topics about which people have strong reactions. In theory, most Americans are fond of individual children and believe that children have a greater claim for help from society and for a share in the resources of the greater society than do many other groups. Although people will articulate these ideas in both public and private conversations, the social situation of many children is not indicative of a country that places special value on children. Children are the age group in American society most likely to live in poverty. Current estimates are that 21.9% of U.S. children live in poverty. Many children live in even worse situations than poverty statistics indicate. Though estimates of the homeless vary, there are probably at least 100,000 children in the United States who go to sleep homeless each night (Oberg, Bryant, & Bach, 1994). Being homeless is a situation that makes it very difficult to attend school, concentrate on schoolwork if school is being attended, or pay attention to overall health concerns, including preventive health issues. Around 10 million children under the age of 18 are without health insurance, meaning that even many families with incomes above the poverty level have difficulty providing health care for their children. The percentage of Americans with employer-based health insurance has decreased over the last 6 years, so that now over 17% of those under age 65 are uninsured. In 13 states, more than a fifth of the population has no health care insurance, and in only one state, Wisconsin, was less than 10% of the nonelderly population uninsured ("Number of Americans," 1995). In 1994, children under 18 accounted for most of the loss of dependents being covered through health insurance plans at the workplace.

These figures, upsetting as they are, are not a creation only of recent decades, especially the figures on poverty. Poverty and poor children have been a major social issue in the United States for the past 100 years, and poor children and families were not unknown in earlier eras as well, although before child labor laws were enacted, children in poor families became workers helping to earn the income of the families at very young ages (working at age 6 or 7 was not unknown as factories began to develop in the United States in the beginning of the 19th century, and leaving school to go to work at ages 12 and 13 was not uncommon at the end of the 19th century). Before that time, poor children often worked beside their parents in farming, if they lived in rural areas, or were apprenticed to learn trades at young ages in cities and larger towns.

Only in the last 100 years has attention been paid to collecting statistics on poverty and to public discussions about basic levels of income required to maintain a family. Poverty was common in colonial America and in the early 19th century but was not considered as much of a general social problem. By the late 1890s and early 1900s ,when the major immigration from European countries was occurring in the United States, social policy reformers became very interested in the large numbers of poor children living in cities. Improving the situation for these children became an interest of some social policy groups, often focused on very specific types of programs such as the creation of settlement houses to work with the poor, especially poor children. Gradually, social policy reforms of the 20th century focused on issues of income disparity, often through discussion of minimum wage laws, and issues of access to social services. More recently, social and health policy reforms have provided access to health insurance to certain social groups, such as the elderly, who used to be an age group (similar to children now) with a higher proportion of poverty than other age groups in the society. In the past, when discussions of welfare policy and helping the needy were debated, poor children were viewed as part of the "worthy poor," those who should not be blamed for their poverty but rather helped to overcome it. In the United States today, one way to generate large numbers of concerned phone calls and donations to special funds is for local television news shows to present special features on a needy child with an unusual disease and with no health insurance, or with health insurance that will not cover an experimental procedure for which treatment is available at a special local hospital or at a hospital in some distant state. Americans are often very generous about donations to help individual children in great need.

This concern about specific individuals and about examples of children with health problems often does not extend to public discussions about the needs of poor, minority children whose mothers are on welfare or public assistance. In fact, Americans often display great inconsistency between how they react to a specific individual in need and how they react to broad categories of individuals. Though generous to the needy individual, especially the needy child, many Americans are also contemptuous of certain groups of the poor or parents who are viewed as caring more about themselves and less about their children. We have developed social myths about certain groups of people, and public discussions and presentations of people in these groups (welfare mothers, "welfare queens," poor children, crack parents, IV drug users) often make assumptions that these parents (especially mothers) care less about their children than do wealthier parents. The same citizens who might generously donate to a local fund to send a child to a hospital halfway around the country to receive emergency surgery may balk at any increase in federal taxes to support welfare programs and Medicaid or any increase in local taxes to support public housing efforts, local programs to provide funds for utility costs, or even increased property taxes to better support public schools.

Though the focus of this book is not on welfare policy or the inconsistencies between American beliefs about individuals versus groups, these issues are one part of understanding how children are viewed in American society today and how their health needs are dealt with by the society overall. One argument of this book is that health needs, although part of the health care system, are increasingly being dealt with by the major social institution in this society that deals with needs of children — the public school systems. In addition, health needs of children (or, for that matter, of other age groups) cannot be completely separated from welfare needs of children. To be healthy, children must be adequately fed and decently housed in a facility with heat or cooling as needed. Recent changes in federal welfare policy that limit the length of time that parents of poor children can receive welfare benefits may have a major impact on the health of children. This may occur even though welfare reform legislation did protect many of the rights of poor children to remain on the Medicaid program and have more access to jointly federal- and state-funded health care services through the Medicaid program.

The focus of this book is the health of children and the role of schools in the health of children. As we change welfare policy in this country, the interaction between all three major social institutions — the health care system, the school system (especially public school systems across the United States), and the welfare system — must be considered. Thus, this book will review material about the health of children both in the past and currently, the roles of schools in society and their relation to the health of children through school health programs in the past, and new models of how schools may deal with the health of children through the growth of school-based clinics and health programs. As part of this, the book will discuss in greater detail one specific state, Arizona, and its efforts to include school-based health care services in some schools. One chapter will focus on the first 2 years of experience of eight projects, all funded by one private foundation in the state, along with a summary of activity in the state through the 1996-97 school year. The last part of this book will link past efforts to protect the health of children with future efforts to deal with the health of children by discussing the impact of recent changes in federal welfare and health policies on children and these changes' possible impact on expanded roles for school services in the overall health of children.

U.S. WELFARE POLICY

Welfare policy in the United States is in a stage of major transition. The major program to provide welfare benefits to children has been Aid to Families with Dependent Children (AFDC) program, earlier known as the (Aid to Dependent Children (ADC) Program. In August 1996, President Clinton signed into law the Personal Responsibility and Work Opportunity Reconciliation Act . This act ended welfare as an entitlement and created a cash welfare block grant called Temporary Assistance for Needy Families (TANF). TANF will replace four existing programs: AFDC, AFDC administration, the Jobs Opportunities and Basic Skills Training (JOBS) Program, and the Emergency Assistance Program. In the fall of 1997, Congress passed the new State Children's Health Insurance Program (SCHIP), which makes available $ 24 billion in funds to states over the next 5 years to help provide health insurance to children. Some of the more specific aspects of the changes will be important factors to consider in the concluding chapter of this book as new approaches for child health policy are discussed. To understand both the immediate past 10 years or so of issues related to child health as well as the initial of the school nursing emphases in this country, however, one must understand the background of the welfare system in this country and more generally how poor and dependent individuals have been viewed. In fact, understanding the background of welfare policy in this country is helpful for understanding both the new changes in federal welfare policy and linkages to child health issues.

Many experts have argued that the root of U.S. policy toward the poor goes back to the British origins of the country and linkages to the English poor-law principles of direct aid for the unemployable, work or imprisonment for the able bodied, and local administration (Handler, 1995). Although outdoor relief was the major thrust in the colonial period and the early years of this country, by the 1820s and 1830s, reformers were advocating poorhouses as the principal form of poor relief. This was part of a broader institutional movement of creating specialized institutions to deal with different social problems: the poorhouse or workhouse for those poor who could work; insane asylums for the mentally ill; separate institutions for the blind, the deaf, and the mute; and orphanages for children too young to be expected to work. Poverty was viewed as presenting a moral challenge to society. Those who were dependent by misfortune did not deserve to be stigmatized in the same manner as the unworthy poor. The work ethic needed to be preserved for adults capable of working (Handler, 1995).

Most histories of welfare in the United States conclude that between 1900 and 1950, both public bureaucracies and private business leaders created an American welfare system that has functioned at both state and federal levels (Berkowitz & McQuaid, 1980; Tomaskovic-Devey, 1988). In 1900, there was no federal level provision for the needs of the poor; instead there were mostly local programs of a charitable nature. Attempts to deal with the poor often focused on moral reform, especially with the children of immigrants, for whom cultural integration into American society was seen as essential (Tomaskovic-Devey, 1988). The welfare system in the United State was a reaction to a rapidly industrializing society in which the role of the federal government initially was also small, with the exception of a few special groups (this has been true of the direct role of the federal government in health care policy as well [Kronenfeld, 1998]. Most of the role of the federal government in welfare provision was either to veterans of the nation's wars or to Indians who were viewed as direct wards of the federal government. The Civil War helped to create additional special categories, with separate institutions for Civil War orphans and separate relief programs for indigent veterans and their families. As Skocpol (1992) has argued, veterans' pensions were a major part of the involvement of the United States government in providing aid to families until the time of the Great Depression and the creation of the major joint federal-state welfare programs under Roosevelt in the 1930s. She has argued that United States historians have underestimated the role of the federal government in welfare provisions because the extensive Civil War pensions have not always been viewed as part of social policy issues. By the end of the 19th century, the Civil War pension program had grown into a massive national income maintenance program through which indigent veterans were morally excused from work. By 1910, the program was ended due to charges of extravagance, corruption, and the vicissitudes of partisan politics (Tomaskovic-Devey, 1988).

Although varied specialized programs to deal with issues of poverty overall and special problems of poor children were created from 1910 to the 1930s, the creation of the U.S. welfare system as we have known it for the past 60 years really began with the Great Depression in the 1930s. Before the federal legislation to create the ADC program, a number of states created programs to provide money to mothers for the care of their children, as long as they were fit and proper mothers. This idea was first endorsed at the federal level in a White House conference in 1909. The first state legislation was passed by Illinois in 1911 and was copied by most of the states by 1925 (Bell, 1965; Handler, 1995; Leff, 1983).

The trauma of the Great Depression, along with the political agitation of the poor at the time for some improved income security, led to the enactment of the basic federal welfare programs (Social Security for the aged and disabled, unemployment insurance, and ADC), even though the Roosevelt administration was most interested in creation of a retirement program (Social Security) and unemployment insurance (Patterson, 1981; Piven & Cloward, 1971). The moral aspect of the primacy of the work ethic remained, with income supports mostly extended to the "deserving poor" such as those too old, too young, or too incapacitated to work.

The ADC program was a grant-in-aid program to the states, with states and local governments administering the program as they thought best, within some fairly broad federal requirements. Through the early 1960s, the program was fairly small, and still predominantly provided funds to widows, most of whom were white, as was the case in the early years of the program. As the civil rights movement grew and the notion of legal rights of welfare recipients became accepted, the numbers of women on welfare increased, as did the ethnic diversity of the women (Handler, 1995). Beginning first in the Kennedy administration in the beginning of the 1960s, with even more expansion under the administrations of Johnson and Nixon, numbers of people on welfare expanded greatly. The Johnson administration started the War on Poverty, with a large increase in the amount of dollars spent on income transfers. This included liberalization of eligibility requirements to include adult members of households with poor children (thus the new title of AFDC), the passage of the Medicare and Medicaid programs to provide health care services to the elderly and the categorically poor, and new programs such as food stamps that helped the poor to extend their incomes to cover basics, such as many food categories. These programs were especially helpful to households with poor children.

Who do we mean when we speak of the poor? One sociologically based definition is that poverty is a social condition characterized by isolation from participation in the culture, most often due to a low level of material resources (Tomaskovic-Devey, 1988). The definition of poverty typically used in empirical studies was originally a nutrition-based estimate of an economy food plan (Orshansky, 1965). This federal poverty measure is the one typically used in official government reports and is a threshold measure, or minimum standard of economic resources needed for a family. This is an example of an absolute measure of poverty, and under this definition, poverty would be eliminated if every family were guaranteed an income above a preset threshold (Aber, Bennett, Conley & Li, 1997). Debate about this official definition continues, with some experts arguing that the measure understates poverty levels because it is not high enough to cover the minimal things now required to be a part of the society and others arguing that it overstates poverty because the value of in-kind contributions to the budget such as food stamps and Medicaid has not been added into the calculations. In contrast, the sociological definition is broader in content and is related to a "relative poverty" type of measure. Such measures are linked to the overall distribution of income and reflect the fact that social inequality per se has negative consequences for individuals regardless of their absolute income level (Aber et al, 1977). Another important aspect of poverty is how long it lasts for any individual or family. Whereas some families are temporarily poor due to a recent divorce or unemployment, others may be poor for a long time and, in the case of children, for their whole childhood. In the United States, this more permanent versus transitory poverty is more characteristic of minorities (Duncan & Rodgers, 1988).

The makeup of the poor population in the United States has been changing. One often commented-upon trend is the feminization of poverty, or the increase in the proportion of poor households that are headed by women and include mostly women and children. In 1967, only 21% of the poor were living in female-headed households with children, whereas this had increased to 36% by 1978. Although the term *feminization* is often used to represent the role of women as heads of more and more poverty-level households, it would be just as accurate to talk about trends of shifting of poverty to children. Whereas during the Depression the elderly were a large age group in which poverty was over represented, the age group now most likely to live in poverty is children. Of the 13.6 million people on welfare in the United States in 1993, 9.2 million were children. About 22 % of all children are living in families below the poverty line. Many other social problems in modern America are associated with living in poverty. Poor children often attend schools of inferior quality, drop out of school at a higher rate in their teenage years, and have more health problems, including higher rates of injury and brain dysfunctions, as well as chronic illnesses such as asthma (Handler, 1995). The connection between poverty and poor health is one of the major reasons that this book is devoting attention to the issue of poverty and welfare changes.

One of the arguments over the last 10 years about growth in numbers of families on welfare has been called the "structural critique of the welfare state." This conservative critique argues that overly generous welfare programs have led to a class of citizens who choose to live in poverty (Murray, 1984; Sanders, 1988; Sowell, 1983). In its essence, this argument posits that public transfers reduce the incentive to work, especially for those who are unlikely to receive salaries much above the minimum wage. Related to this argument is a general dissatisfaction with public welfare because of the belief that taxes were raised, especially between the mid-1960s and mid-1980s, in order to fund an overly generous welfare system. Without reviewing in detail all of the evidence as to the accuracy of these arguments (and there is conflicting evidence depending on the time periods used and the specific figures used), the consensus about welfare reform for almost 30 years has been that able-bodied welfare recipients should work (Handler, 1995). How this notion has meshed with the situation of mothers of children is more complex, for societal norms have been shifting from a belief that mothers should stay at home, at least with younger children if not with all children, to greater public acceptance of mothers working, even with very young children.

Work requirements for welfare recipients began as a federal concern with the work incentive (WIN) program in 1967 and are a major push of the new Clinton administration welfare reforms. As some social critics and welfare experts have pointed out, work requirements for welfare recipients first became a major part of public discussion in 1967, a year by which a growing number of AFDC recipients were never married and African Americans had become a larger proportion of the AFDC recipients (Handler, 1995). Before this point, the official position of those who studied welfare and the welfare bureaucracy, as well as most politicians, was that families would become self-supporting through social services. Disillusionment with this position grew through the 1960s as welfare rolls increased and costs grew, resulting in the WIN program. Though in theory, WIN required adults over age 16, including mothers, to register with state employment services for training and employment, options for exemptions were possible, and by 1971, only 24% of welfare recipients were considered "appropriate for referral" to the employment service (Handler & Hasenfeld, 1991). Though much of the public believed that unmarried mothers should be able to provide for their children without public help, the conflicting belief that young mothers should be home with children helped to retain large numbers of exemptions from WIN-type requirements in this time period. Most attempts to change welfare either failed or had only symbolic impact. Nixon's Family Assistance Plan, which would have greatly expanded incentives for work, was defeated in Congress. A major effort by President Carter that contained many features of the recently enacted welfare reform and included a major push for the "able-bodied" to work also failed to pass Congress.

The Reagan administration focused on welfare reform and had greater success than some previous administrations in getting some of the proposed changes passed. The reforms had a more severe impact on women and children, despite general American values that reject increased impoverishment for children (Gotsch-Thompson, 1988). The Reagan administration was able to capitalize on the idea that business should gain more freedoms and that the welfare state should be diminished due to concerns of welfare fraud, without sounding as if children and the elderly would be penalized, given that much of the administration's public rhetoric discussed the importance of retaining the safety net for the truly needy (Gotsch-Thompson, 1988). States were given greater flexibility for welfare reforms, and over half of the states adopted work requirements as demonstration projects.

The Personal Responsibility and Work Opportunity Reconciliation Act of 1996 imposes a 5-year limit on most families' benefits and will gradually be implemented in states. The success at passing this legislation followed a campaign promise of Clinton's that he would "end welfare as we know it." The Republican Contract With America that led to the election of a Republican-controlled Congress in the 1994 elections had also announced that welfare reform was a major goal, with a focus on "family values" and correcting the moral decline of American society and a designation of welfare as the public policy most destructive of the American family (Watts, 1997). The new law places a cap on federal funding for welfare programs (the new TANF) through the year 2002, with each state receiving its allocation through a block grant to the state, with a provision for less funding if a state does not meet its federally mandated work participation rates. This new law partially reflects the changing notions about women and work. As over half of mothers of children under age 6 are now in the labor force, a welfare system that protects the rights of mothers to remain at home with children and out of the labor force is less and less acceptable politically. Further discussion of this law and its possible impacts on child health and welfare will be discussed in more detail in Chapter 6, after other aspects of child health and child health policy have been discussed. Federal welfare policy provides the major context for many aspects of life for poor children in the United States. The health of children is greatly influenced by welfare policy, as well as by changes in the health care system, health policy, and school health issues.

SCHOOLS AND HEALTH CARE

This first chapter has focused on the interactions between three major societal institutions that deal with children: the health care delivery system, the education system, and the welfare system. Most of the chapter has discussed the welfare system in the United States, especially as it relates to children and to changes in mandatory work requirements for parents. The rest of the book will focus on health care and schools and the interaction between those two social institutions, with some focus again at the end of the book on broader social policy issues, including changes in the welfare system in the United States. Chapter 2 will focus on school health programs, including a review of the initial premises behind the creation of school health programs in the United States and how they have developed over the last century. This is linked to changes in the health status of children, and one section will review some historical material on the health of children. Issues about the economy and how it affects families, as well as policy about the delivery of health care services and health education programs, will be discussed briefly in this chapter.

Chapter 3 will review material on the health status of children in the United States currently, along with some discussion of child health in other countries. Understanding some of the major issues in child health status is necessary before the new role of schools in helping to improve the health status of children can be discussed.

Chapter 4 will discuss the growth of expanded school health programs. It will discuss a number of the earlier models of this approach and describe the differences between school-based health centers and school-linked health centers. This chapter will also include some discussion of differences between programs aimed at younger children and those aimed at adolescents and the different receptions to programs depending on the age-group of children who are the intended recipients of services.

This book originated from my experience of several decades with preventive health programs and with child safety research and is also related to my interests in the overall topics of child health and health care policy. More specifically, this book started with the evaluation of what began as six quite different projects relating to the provision of health care to children in six school districts within Arizona in the fall of 1993 (and expanded the next year to nine projects), all funded by a large private health-oriented foundation in the state, the Flinn Foundation.

Though all evaluation projects are unique, this evaluation dealt with a changing set of projects, changing timetables within each project, and changing goals of a number of the projects. Moreover, the diversity of the projects triggered interests in many varied aspects of child health and school health, leading to the focus of this book. Two of the initial projects focused on high school students and adolescent health-related issues, including behavioral aspects of health as well as physical aspects; three focused on provision of some health care services at the school site during regular school times and hoped to see improvements in child health and in prevention of problems such as might be indicated by reductions in absenteeism from school. One project focused more on the use of the school as a convenient site for the provision of some basic health screening, immunization, and eligibility determination and was not conducted during school hours, but focused on innovative uses of the school setting to provider broader sets of health and welfare services to school-age children and their parents. A year later, several additional school-based health projects in Arizona were also funded by the same foundation and became part of an evaluation effort. A more detailed examination of the experiences of these projects and ongoing efforts in Arizona is presented in Chapter 5.

The concluding chapter of the book, Chapter 6, integrates the material on child health, the past efforts of school health programs, and the experiences of the last decade in the creation of school-based clinics, the creation of managed-care Medicaid programs, and welfare and child health care reform in the United States to discuss future issues in child health and ways in which extended school health programs may be included in new programs to deal with the health of children.

CHAPTER 2

HISTORY OF CHILD HEALTH AND SCHOOL HEALTH PROGRAMS

Background and Current Roles of School Health Programs

Concern with child health is not a new idea. This chapter will begin with documentation that creating a role for schools in improving the health of children is also not a new idea, although the direct provision of services for all types of care for children in a school setting is a newer approach. The role that schools can play in the health of children is great because, from age 5 or 6 on, children spend a large proportion of their waking hours in a school setting. Schools can have an influence on health through the practices they present, through direct education programs, and, more recently, through the provision of health care services to children. The school is one of the few environments in our society in which the state (government) can influence citizens directly in large numbers, and for this reason alone, as well as because participation in public schools is one of the most commonly shared experiences in the society, schools are a useful place to educate children about health and to check for health care needs (Pickett & Hanlon, 1990).

The first section of this chapter will review the historical development of school health nursing and the concern about health for children in a school setting, along with historical material on child health. The second section will discuss various types of programs that are typically included in schools as part of the services of the school nurse. The third section addresses the issue of other ways in which health needs are addressed in schools, especially in elementary schools; the focus here is on school health education programs. By reviewing how health concerns in the school have been handled in the past and are currently handled through more traditional programs of school nursing and school health education, this chapter provides important background information for a more detailed look at the health of children today and at how models of delivery of health care services in schools and the development of school-based clinics and health care centers can help to improve the health of children now and in the future.

HISTORICAL BACKGROUND ON CHILDREN'S HEALTH AND SCHOOL HEALTH PROGRAMS

More detailed professional concern with child health, especially within the schools, begins with reform movements at the beginning of the 20th century in the United States and actually in a similar time period in some other countries, such as the United Kingdom (While & Barriball, 1993). This section of the chapter reviews the historical material about the health of children and the creation of school health programs as a way to deal with child health concerns. It also connects this view of child health and school health programs to broader social concerns at the time. Finally, it addresses the linkages between the developments of nursing, social work, and public school teaching and how these professions have or have not worked together to deal with the health care needs of children in public schools.

The health of children today is enormously better than in the past. The mortality rate for children has improved by nearly 10-fold since the beginning of the 20th century, dropping from roughly 4 per 1,000 to less than 0.5 (Pickett & Hanlon, 1990). The reduction is mostly due to the decline in deaths from communicable diseases. In 1900, diphtheria was the leading cause of death for children from ages 5 to 14, followed by non-motor-vehicle accidents, pneumonia and influenza, and tuberculosis. Diphtheria and tuberculosis as causes of death are largely gone, and non-motor-vehicle unintentional injuries have declined, primarily because of environmental factors such as improved building codes and housing codes, although deaths from motor vehicle injuries are now the most common cause of death in children in this age group.

One of the most commonly used measures of health status is the infant mortality rate, or the number of deaths that occur in the first year of life, generally stated per 1,000 births. In the late 19th century in the United States, about 200 of every 1,000 children born alive would die before the age of 1. The major causes of death for these children were dysentery, pneumonia, measles, diphtheria and whooping cough. By 1925, the infant mortality rate was 75, a substantial reduction. For 1993, the infant mortality rate was 8.3. As compared to 100 years ago, we now have vaccinations for measles, diphtheria, and whooping cough, so that generally there are no infant deaths due to these causes. Improved sanitation, pasteurization of milk, and better medications (such as penicillin, other related drugs and other drugs to deal with pneumonia) have all reduced the numbers of deaths from other causes to very small numbers.

If we try to summarize the major achievements in child health over the past century, control of infectious or communicable diseases has been one major area of accomplishment (Behrman, 1996). First, vaccines were developed for such diseases as whooping cough and tetanus. In the 1950s, polio, which was a major infectious disease that led to lifelong disability if not death and was a major fear among parents from the 1930s through the early 1950s, was controlled by a new vaccination. More recently, other remaining common childhood diseases such as measles, which still caused child deaths before the development of the vaccine, have been controlled. In the last few years, even some of the less serious childhood diseases in terms of death, such as chicken pox, are now controllable by vaccines. Though children did not die from chicken pox, it did sometimes leave disfiguring marks on the skin and was problematic for working parents, since someone had to be home with the sick child, often for a week or longer.

In addition to control of infectious diseases, better understanding of nutrition and better overall public health have had a major impact in improving morbidity and mortality for children. Better nutrition has generally eliminated such problems as goiters and rickets. Better overall environments and sanitation have controlled health problems such as hookworm and lessened greatly the impact of such problems as dysentery and dehydration.

The early public health movement focused on issues such as adequate food and shelter and proper ventilation in growing tenements in major cities. In the period after the Civil War, sanitary facilities and sewers were undeveloped, with sewage often disposed of in streets. Diarrhea and gastrointestinal disorders were common, as was bronchitis. These problems were found not only in private homes and apartments but even in special institutions designed to care for children, such as the New York City Foundling Home. In fact, often the worst overall environments for young children were such institutions. In 1881, nearly four times as many infants died in the New York City Foundling Home as in better institutions outside the city (King, 1993).

Some social reformers began to call the 20th century the century of the child and were able to attract growing attention to the health of children. Science formed the foundation for the 20th century medical care of children, and the Children's Bureau Publication of a booklet on infant care became a major method of teaching mothers about safe milk, the importance of immunization, and the importance of hydration (keeping fluids down) for sick children. By 1921, over 1.5 million copies of this pamphlet had been distributed (King, 1993). By the 1920s, the health of American children had improved, as indicated by the large reduction in the infant mortality rate from the turn of the century to 1925. By the 1920s, improved living conditions, wide-scale vaccination, better nutrition, improved prenatal and maternal health care, and specific health reforms such as pasteurization of milk supplies meant that many fewer children died from common diseases of childhood. Further improvement came in the middle of the 20th century with the introduction of antibacterial chemicals and antibiotic agents. Because of these improvements, pediatric medicine now spends much of its time on chronic conditions (Behrman, 1996; King, 1993). This quick review of the past health of children links to the concerns that educators and nurses had about the health of school-age children 100 years ago, and the beginning of school health programs.

The health of school-age children and especially the health of poorer children have been a concern within the public health, health education, nursing, and health services community for almost 100 years, beginning during the era of heavy immigration into the major U.S. cities at the turn of the 19th century into the 20th century (Hawkins, Hayes, & Corliss, 1994; Pollitt, 1994). The crowded living conditions, poverty, and high rates of morbidity and mortality due to communicable infectious diseases such as tuberculosis, diphtheria, and whooping cough were major concerns of public health nursing at that time. One of the founders of modern nursing in the United States and a person also often recognized as the first school nurse in the United States was Lillian Ward. She was an energetic public health nurse and social reformer who graduated from the New York Hospital School of Nursing in 1891 (Pollitt, 1994). Wald moved to the East Side of New York City in 1892 and founded what became known as the Henry Street Settlement. The nurses that were part of her group not only provided home health services but started the first special education programs, established the first playgrounds in the United States, developed the idea of "fresh-air" camps in the summer for inner-city children, and became interested in all aspects of the lives of the people in their areas. In this time period, women active in settlement houses often combined what are today two separate professional roles: public health nurse and social worker. Back then, the professional demarcations were less clear.

In addition to its important role as the largest U.S. city and the city that was the route of entry for most immigrants to the United States, New York City was one of the first cities to have a mandatory school attendance law. The large number of immigrant children in the schools, due to both the city's role in immigration and the mandatory attendance law, meant that conditions of children related to poor sanitation, such as ringworm, impetigo, conjunctivitis, and head lice, were major problems in many schools in New York City. To deal with this, in 1897, the New York City Department of Health hired 150 doctors for an hour a day to inspect poor children. Students with contagious conditions were sent home (Pollitt, 1994). This exclusionary program was not that successful. Among the reasons for lack of success were that no treatments were given to the children, the children remained in the neighborhood to play with children in school and thus were able to reinfect them, and some teachers resisted the inspections because they felt it was more important for children to remain in school and be able to receive an education than it was to deal with the diseases. Advice was sought from the Henry Street nurses about how to deal with these problems, and they suggested using a nurse to treat the children in the schools and having a school-based nurse available to help parents understand the problems and help them learn how to create more healthful conditions in their home.

Four schools with the greatest number of exclusions were chosen as sites for a month-long experiment with having nurses in the schools that was later deemed successful. Thus, school nursing developed as an outgrowth of the public health movement, with the first school nurse employed by the New York City Schools in 1902 (Passarelli, 1994). By 1903, the number of children excluded from classes for health reasons dropped by 90% due to the presence of the nurses. By then, 25 registered nurses were employed in 125 public schools in New York City (Pollitt, 1994). In its beginnings, school nursing included more detailed examinations of some children and treatments for disease, with records showing nurses treating 980,637 cases of contagion among 93,000 schoolchildren in 1905 in New York City. Over 40,000 visits to tenements were held to meet with parents. By 1914, New York City was employing 374 school nurses. Although the roles of these nurses have changed over the years, their early beginnings were tied both to public health and to actual delivery of health care services, both of which factors would also be important in the growth of school-based clinics.

After the success in New York, other places also began programs of school nursing. The Los Angeles Board of Health appointed its first school nurse in 1905, followed by Boston in 1905 and Philadelphia in 1908 (Pollitt, 1994). Interestingly, school health services were established in other countries around the same time. The school health service in Great Britain was established in 1908, and school health nurses there worked as assistants to school medical officers, spending most of their time screening for infectious and contagious diseases and treating minor health problems (Wile & Barriball, 1993).

As the innovation spread, specifics of what school nursing entailed and how schools should become involved in health were also clarified in more states. In 1910, New Jersey became the first state to enact a statute for the general physical examination of schoolchildren. These early evaluations emphasized remediable conditions, such as dental caries, visual loss, hearing difficulties, postural defects, and other preventable or readily treated ailments (King, 1993). These efforts were adopted by other states, and large numbers of health problems were found, especially among poorer children.

The growth of school health was occurring at the same time that pediatrics was becoming a recognized specialty within medicine and that interest in the health of children was growing. The section in the American Medical Association that focused on diseases of children was established in 1880. The American Pediatric Society was formed in 1888. Although there was controversy in the emerging field of pediatrics about whether appropriate care for children needed to include broader social issues as well, by the early 20th century, most pediatricians supported some emphasis on the social basis of children's health.

Concerns about health of children in schools grew out of concerns about infectious diseases and their spread and the eras increasing emphasis on cleanliness, based on a beginning understanding of the germ theory of disease. It was in this era that public efforts began to control flies, to convince people to wash their hands, and to engage in sanitary disposal of wastes. Use of cow milk as food for infants began to grow in the 1890s, but for it to be safe for children, the purity of the milk supply had to be ensured. In 1916, less than 1% of the nation's total milk supply was certified as pure (King, 1993). Given these levels of knowledge and public practice, some focus on child health was needed. From its origins in public health concerns, school nursing began with a model for practice that was considerably more independent than became the case in later years (Hawkins et al., 1994).

The health of school-age children became the initial focus of the Child Health Organization, founded in 1917 by Emmett Holt, the author of the most influential text at the time on diseases of infancy and childhood. This organization encouraged teachers to promote the health of their pupils and urged the creation of school programs for nutrition, including free lunches for poor children (King, 1993). They also encouraged the study of the health of schoolchildren. In addition, a goal of the organization became the education of schoolchildren about health so that they could be healthier as adults and bring improved knowledge into their own families. A separate organization focused on infant health had been founded in 1908, first called the American Association for the Study and Prevention of Infant Health and eventually renamed the American Child Hygiene Association. These types of organizations led to more public attention and interest in child health and thus a more important role for schools in improving the health status of children.

The Child Health Organization merged with the American Child Hygiene Association in 1922, taking the name of the American Child Health Association (ACHA). That organization promoted a Child's Bill of Rights at the initial meeting and advanced political solutions for the problem of children's health. As part of its effort to obtain more information, it conducted a survey of health conditions in 86 American cities along with a survey of milk supplies from 650 cities in 30 states. As an illustration of the widespread nature of problems found, nearly half of the milk supplies were contaminated, and 85% were delivered without ice or refrigeration (King, 1993). At about the same time, a Children's Bureau study of children in rural Kentucky conducted in 1922 found dental caries and tonsil problems for about three quarters of the children examined (Roberts, 1922). Similar rates of problems were found in New York City (King, 1993). The gathering of data on problems helped to create further discussion about the need to improve child health.

The most important federal institution for promoting the health of children in the first half of the 20th century was the Children's Bureau, established in 1912, with Julie Lathrop, an associate of Jane Addams, as its first director. Despite controversy over its founding, due to both opposition over the expenditure of federal funds on the problems of maternal and child health and a belief by many that these types of problems were best handled at home, the bureau filled an important void. Its early focus was on infant mortality, but the pursuit of broader goals led to increased attention at the state and municipal level to the problems of the health of children and led major cities such as New York to establish their own children's bureaus to deal with more specialized local problems. Kansas set up the first state-level bureau in 1915 and encouraged children's health fairs as well as a focus on maternal and infant health (King, 1993). The activities of states were further encouraged by the passage of the Sheppard-Towner Act in 1921. This act increased funds for many infant and child health programs, especially for educational programs. The act did not survive changing norms about the role of government and the opposition of the American Medical Association, however, and it was not renewed in 1929 (Kronenfeld & Whicker, 1984).

The Depression in the 1930s and World War II in the 1940s were periods of rapid social change, ultimately leading to less emphasis on state and federal funding for school-related health services as more crucial needs of families and children became emphasized. Like the earlier waves of immigration, the widespread poverty of the Depression initially increased the need for attention to the health of children within the public schools of the nation. In this time period, children's health care became more institutionalized overall, and physicians became stronger spokespersons for children's health, but with a focus more on individual children and private health care than on the community and schools as a place in which children congregate. The Depression did lead to increased recognition that poverty was the root cause of many of the health care problems of children and that the health care of children required more than the treatment of sick children and the dispensing of medications. During this time period, immunization programs and school physical examinations helped to provide some preventive care for all children (King, 1993). World War II brought great demand overall for nurses, as many were needed by the armed forces. Communities struggled to meet the demands of war and the needs of the civilian population, including schoolchildren (Hawkins et al., 1994). School health nursing experienced little growth during World War II.

As had happened at the end of World War I, the high rejection rates of recruits to the military due to health problems in World War II provided evidence that the health of many children was not adequate. Childhood nutrition was promoted by the passage of the National School Lunch Act in 1946 (42 §1751). At the Mid-Century White House Conference on Children and Youth, there was discussion of the need to develop in children the mental, emotional, and spiritual qualities essential to individual happiness. Proposed efforts focused on the whole child and were expanded to include handicapped children. One of the major outcomes from this conference was the establishment of statewide programs for handicapped children.

Development of better immunizations led to more control of infectious diseases, as did hard work in earlier decades of school nursing and public health that had led to better control of communicable conditions such as impetigo and ringworm (Hawkins et al., 1994). More attention was placed on health screenings, including hearing and vision screening. These were major foci in the more affluent 1950s.

By the 1960s, school health nursing in most communities was quite separate from public health nursing. In later chapters, the growth of school-based clinics and a renewed emphasis on the role of the school in the health of children will be explored. One way to conceptualize the history of school nursing is as a movement from a public health model to a heavily school-based model. The new trends may indicate renewed interest in the relation of school health concerns to overall community health.

From the 1960s to the present, school nurses and pediatricians have addressed a variety of child health issues, from child abuse to problems such as lead poisoning and child safety. A very important program for the health and nutrition of children, the Special Supplemental Food Program for Women, Infants and Children (WIC) was passed in 1975. Most of these efforts, however, did not single out schools as a site for health efforts, although school health examinations and the incorporation of health education content into curriculums (especially at the elementary level) have continued.

THE SCHOOL NURSE

One debate that has continued from the beginning of use of nurses in schools is whether school health services should be minimal activities designed to facilitate learning or whether they should be more comprehensive (Passarelli, 1994; Pickett & Hanlon, 1990). A related issue, addressed in the next section, is the role of school nurses in education of children about health. As one recent article on the outlook of school health nursing in the future asked, "Where does the field of school health nursing see itself on the continuum between illness and injury related roles and the pro-active, health promoting and preserving functions of school health nursing?" (Salmon, 1994, p. 137). There are also controversies over the level of education a school nurse needs and who besides registered nurses (RNs) should be able to provide school health services. A still more recent issue is the increasing expectation that school nurses be able to deal with behavioral health problems and whether it is appropriate for school nurses to add behavioral health care to the other required tasks.

Numbers of school nurses have not increased at the same rate as the school-age population. Today, about 30,000 school nurses in 110,000 elementary and secondary schools are responsible for meeting the health needs of over 42 million students, a ratio of one nurse to every 1,400 students (Bradley, 1997; "Exploring National Issues," 1996; Bradley, 1997). Obviously, the typical school nurse is not seeing most students on even an irregular basis. This situation is not changing much. In a recent survey of school districts, most (75%) had not changed the size of their nursing staff over the past 3 years (Fryer & Igoe, 1995). The ratio of school nurses to students actually varies greatly by state, ranging from 1 nurse per 486 students in New Hampshire up to 1 nurse per 10,814 students in Tennessee. Health services facilities are not available in about 32% of all middle/junior and senior high schools (Small et al., 1995).

As evidence that numbers of school nurses may actually matter for the health of children in a given area, one study rank-ordered states by the ratio of students to nurses and looked at the correlation between this rank order and ranking of the states on child well-being indices (Fryer & Igoe, 1995). Children did appear to be better off in states with more school nurses, with a correlation of .486 between the two rankings.

How might the presence of school nurses affect student health? The answer lies in the activities undertaken by a typical school nurse. At a minimum, most school health nurses provide some combination of acute, chronic, episodic, and emergency health care (Passarelli, 1994). A recent description of a typical day for a school nurse in one article discussing the trends for the future of school nursing listed the following activities:

> assessment of abdominal pain, skin rashes, headaches and head injuries, counseling students regarding issues of sexuality, drug use or AIDS, education and supervision of school personnel regarding management of seizures in the classroom, assessment of a possible child abuse situation, management of anaphylaxis in a student or staff member and support of a child whose father was recently killed. (Passarelli, 1994, pp. 141-142)

Activities and Services of School Nurses

Some roles for school nurses are similar across the country. All states require children to be immunized against certain communicable diseases, and in many school districts, school nurses have the mostly administrative function of keeping immunization records for each child (as well as other health records) and being sure that immunizations are up to date. Although this may seem a small task, immunization of children is one of the most critical aspects of overall community health. In a 1994 study of state and district health education policies in the Unites States, 99.7% of middle/junior and senior high schools maintained immunization records on file for each student, and over 80% kept medical information forms, medical emergency forms, screening records, and medication administration directions (Small et al., 1995). Most public schools perform this task fairly efficiently, although one recent study in two selected school districts in the Pittsburgh area found that a significant number of children were lacking recommended immunizations for the age at entry to school, despite a recent physician visit (Bradford, Heald, Benedum & Petrie, 1996). Though these types of special studies indicate the need for continued vigilance regarding immunization status, especially within the elementary schools, the major push in immunization efforts today is to lower the attainment of complete immunizations to the age of 2, rather than waiting for children to begin school ("Status Report," 1997).

During the 1940s and 1950s, a major task for school nurses was customarily the examination of every schoolchild every year. Over time, this practice became viewed as both inefficient and ineffective because so many children had to be examined that mostly cursory attention was paid to most children. The administrative and record-keeping aspect of this task was major, however, leaving the school nurse little time for other activities. As the practice of an overall examination for each child has declined, what has remained as a task for the school nurse is screening for major health problems and for such problems as vision and hearing defects. These types of screening programs, which fit within a minimalist general philosophy that school health services should ensure that a child is in the condition to learn and that uncorrected hearing and vision defects hinder the attainment of the school's educational goals, are now common in many elementary schools. Even 80% of middle/junior high schools in a recent survey conducted health screening activities, especially vision and hearing screening (Small et al., 1995).

Screening, especially vision screening, is an important task in schools because abnormal visual acuity is the most common chronic condition in children who live in industrialized nations (Angle & Wissman, 1980; Yawn, Lydick, Epstein & Jacobsen, 1996). Most schools now conduct either yearly or biyearly screenings for visual acuity. One recent study that followed a population-based cohort of children entering kindergarten in a 3-year period found that overall, 28% of children had at least one abnormal school vision screening test (Yawn et al., 1996). Overall, 92% of children referred for further testing after the screening process actually received evaluation from an eye professional, indicating the importance of the screening in leading to recognition and correction of the problem. School vision screening provided the first indication of abnormal visual acuity in 76% of the children in the cohort, a finding that underscores the importance of school screening. Most children identified by the school screening as having a vision problem had the problem confirmed by the visit to the eye care professional (85% on the first visit and 98% by age 18), a further indication that school screening is a low-cost method of identification of visual problems, one that does not cause parents to obtain unnecessary eye services. This study also found that boys' vision problems seem to peak at a later age than girls', so that the common practice of curtailing vision screenings at age 13 or seventh grade may not be a good practice.

One major role of school nurses is first aid and the evaluation of sick students. These are very common services in schools, and even if there is no school nurse available, someone in the school must perform them. In one study of middle/junior high schools and high schools, first aid was provided in 98%. Often people besides the school nurse provide first aid, including classroom teachers, secretaries, and health aides. In about half of the schools, if first aid is provided by someone other than a nurse, certification by the Red Cross or a similar agency is required (Small et al., 1995). If a nurse is available, the task of evaluating whether a student should be sent home is generally performed by the nurse.

As concern about issues such as child abuse has grown and as legal reporting requirements have been instituted in most states, the legal responsibility for teachers and especially for school nurses to report suspected cases of child abuse has created a new task for school nurses, one that places the nurse in opposition to the parents if suspected child abuse is reported. Identification of violence-related injuries treated in the school setting has been listed as one of the five important benchmarks for school nurses to establish (Igoe, 1994).

Another change in the role of school nurses began with the passage of Public Law 94-142 (20 USC 1401), the Education of All Handicapped Children Act, in 1975. This law made school nurses responsible for meeting the health needs of physically and mentally disabled students as they were mainstreamed into schools ("Exploring National Issues," 1996). Also, the Rehabilitation Act of 1973 (29 §701) has mandated educational and support service protection for individuals with disabilities. In New York City before 1980, many children with serious physical handicaps were educated in special Public Centers for Multiply Handicapped Children. By September 1994, 180 nurses were employed by the board of education to care for children in kindergarten through 12th grade who now attended regular public schools as part of satisfying the "least restrictive environment" provisions of these laws. The children covered by the laws included multiply handicapped children as well as those who were survivors of advanced pediatric technology largely unavailable and possibly unforseen when the laws were originally passed (Lipper, Farr, Marchese, Palfrey, & Darby, 1997).

Related to these laws, as well as to the growth of behavioral health diagnoses among younger children, is the increase in tasks for school health nurses that involve dealing with either children with behavioral health problems who may require medication during the school day to help deal with these problems or children with chronic health problems. Today, any given school is likely to contain some students with serious chronic health problems that have complicated management schedules (Williams & McCarthy, 1995), as well as a large number of children with less severe but serious health problems, such as asthma, one of the most rapidly increasing health problems among school-age children, that may require medication during the day. In one study of middle and high schools, about 80% of schools allowed students to carry medications if they were part of a prescribed regimen. Inhalers were the medication most frequently carried by the children themselves (Small et al., 1995).

As part of both the growth in the numbers of schoolchildren with chronic health problems and behavioral health problems, use of both prescription and nonprescription medications has increased among children (Francis, Hemmat, Treolar, & Yarandi, 1996). In one study about use of medications in 36 public schools and six private school, children received drugs in 31 different drug categories. Medications ranged from over the counter to the most commonly used drug, methylphenidate HCL (better known by its trademark name of Ritalin). The other major categories of drugs used were bronchodilators, analgesics, antihypertensives, anticonvulsives, antiinfectives, and antidepressants. About 3.5% of the sampled school population received 5,101 doses of medication while in school. The number of boys taking medications was 2.5 times higher than the number of girls, partially because of higher rates of use of drugs for behavioral health problems for boys. Most sources agree that attention deficit hyperactivity disorder (ADHD) is more prevalent in boys than girls (Arnold & Jensen, 1995). The single most frequently used drug in schools in this survey was methylphenidate for ADHD (Francis et al., 1996). In this study, 3% of students were taking this one medication, a figure in line with the findings of other studies (Arnold & Jensen, 1995; Costello, 1989; Francis et al., 1996).

Licensure, Level of Provider, and Legal and Administrative Issues

The National Association of School Nurses has argued that a baccalaureate degree from an accredited college or university should be the minimum preparation for entry into school nursing. This is not a new recommendation; throughout the history of school nursing, a baccalaureate education with additional preparation in health education has been suggested for school nurses (Passarelli, 1994). Many schools, however, have often simply required that a nurse hold a RN license. In the past, this could be obtained through a 4-year degree program, a 3-year hospital program, or a 2-year associate degree program in a community college. Most new nurses today hold either a 2-year or a 4-year degree, since hospital training programs have largely disappeared. About half of school nurses hold a baccalaureate degree, mostly in nursing (Bradley, 1997). In a few states, credentialing as a school nurse requires a fifth year of college work that may include health education, pedagogy and teaching strategies.

Only a few states require a fifth year of training in addition to a degree, and not all districts follow the recommendation that school nurses have a BS degree. More recent debate, however, is not so much over whether an RN from a 2-year AA degree program in nursing is acceptable as over the use of nursing assistants. In 1995, only 16 states required that school health services be provided by a registered professional nurse, and only two states had mandated minimum student-to-nurse ratios ("The State of School Nursing Today," 1995). In 1993, the American Nurses Association's *Standards of Clinical Nursing Practice* were applied to the specialty of school nursing (Bradley, 1997; Proctor, Lordi & Zeiger, 1993). In 1996, a position paper about the delegation of school health services to unlicenced assistive personnel was issued (National Association of State School Nurse Consultants, 1996). It argued, first, that to benefit from educational programs and to maximize energy for learning, students with chronic health problems must maintain their health at an optimal level and that they can best do this by having access to health care services provided by RNs, and qualified unlicenced assistive personnel (UAPs), to whom RNs delegate care. Second, the paper argued that safe delegation requires that individualized student health plans be developed by the RN in collaboration with the student, family health care providers, and the school team. Third, it argued that the RN must use professional judgment to decide which student care activities may be delegated, as framed by the state nursing practice acts and national standards of nursing.

Who UAPs are may vary from district to district. Only a limited number of states certify health assistants. In many, no preservice training programs are required, although many districts do try to run their own inservice programs for these personnel (Fryer & Igoe, 1995). UAPs have different titles in different states, including that of school health aide and school health assistant. In some places, classroom aides and secretaries may serve partially as school health aides also.

In one nationwide survey of a systematic random sample of school districts, most school districts relied heavily on nursing personnel for technically involved clinical services but often employed health assistants to administer medications and basic first aid (Fryer & Igoe, 1996). Most districts that participated in the survey had not used the health assistants to replace RNs, with only 9% of districts surveyed reporting a cut in RN employment due to the use of aides. As noted in the previous section, which discusses growing use of medications in schools, use of all types of medications has been increasing. Similarly, the number of families in which both parents work, leaving no one easily available to come and pick up a sick child, has also been increasing. This has led parents to support less restrictive school policies about the administration of medications. Whereas 20 years ago, many schools would not administer even minor pain medication such as aspirins to children, most schools now will obtain this permission as part of a routine form that parents complete at the beginning of the year. Though nurses agree that the ideal situation would be the administration of drugs by RNs, the reality is that medications are often given by nonhealth personnel. In that setting, a paraprofessional under the supervision of the nurse is a better solution than the secretary or a classroom aide (Francis et al., 1996). In one study of middle/junior high schools and high schools, 64% allowed secretaries to administer some medications, and 19% allowed teachers to do so (Small et al., 1995). About a quarter of high schools allow students to self-administer drugs, although drug control policies in some districts have led to controversies over students carrying common medications such as aspirin or cold pills in their materials during the school day, resulting in some recent cases that have received national publicity in which students were suspended from schools for having such remedies as aspirin in their purses or backpacks.

Administration and supervision of school nurses have often been complicated because administrative structures of school systems differ greatly from those of health care systems ("The State of School Nursing Today," 1995). School nursing services are often directed by non-health-care personnel, and the school nurse is often not directly accountable to a nursing supervisor. One 1991 survey found that only 60% of school districts with an identifiable school health program reported the major academic discipline of the administrator of school nursing to be nursing ("The State of School Nursing Today," 1995). The new laws for students with chronic health problems and disabilities have increased the complexity of the tasks that the school nurse may be expected to perform (Harrison, Faircloth, & Yaryan, 1995). One recent piece of legislation is Public Law 100-407 (29 USC 2201), which addresses the need for assistive technologies in the provision of services to children with disabilities. Nurses in school settings now have the legal responsibility to be aware of the use and management of these technologies in the school setting. One important issue is professional liability. Given the increased numbers of students in the school population who are medically fragile, the school nurse is subject to increased levels of liability. School systems may need to increase their liability coverages for nurses and perhaps to review the responsibilities of unlicenced personnel in these more complicated situations. At this point, some boundaries are not clear, and probably case law resulting from litigation will determine the real limits (Harrison et al., 1995).

HEALTH EDUCATION PROGRAMS IN THE SCHOOLS

In the early years of school health nursing, education of both parents and students was another important activity for the school nurse. As more programs of formal health education have developed, the tasks of the nurse generally have focused more on activities around screening and treatment of sick children than ON a formal educational role. One of the classic definitions of school health responsibilities discusses three different goals: health services, health education, and a healthful school environment (Igoe, 1994). The preceding section has discussed the more traditional health services aspects of school nursing, and Chapters 4 and 5 will focus in more detail on expanded models of school health services. The rest of this chapter focuses on delivery of the other two components, with more emphasis on health education. One recent expanded definition of a comprehensive school health program describes eight interactive components: health education, physical education and other physical activities, health services, food services, school counseling and social services, integrated school and community efforts, faculty and staff health promotion, and the school environment (Kahn et al., 1995). One of the 10 standards for school nursing practice encompasses health education. It states that the school nurse assists students, families, and the school community to achieve optimal levels of wellness through appropriately designed and delivered health education (Bradley, 1997). Often a distinction has been made between one-on-one health education, done either as a nursing intervention or as part of health counseling, and more group-oriented approaches (Bradley, 1997). Many of the new school-based clinics view health counseling as important, but this section will focus more on other types of health education efforts that are less oriented to a particular student or client. In many schools, the nurse may support classroom-based health education by providing inservice programming for teachers and acting as a consultant to health teachers (Bradley, 1997). Less formally, school nurses also may share materials from their own health-oriented libraries with teachers in the school.

The federal government has played a number of important roles in helping to develop school health efforts, as have professional groups and some private corporations. Early efforts at development of comprehensive school health education programs and curricula were begun in New York State under Rockefeller as governor. The National Education Association was the sponsor of the School Health Education Study in the early 1960s (Cortese, 1993). This study, which presented results of a nationwide survey of instructional processes, showed that many topics were being avoided by schools. This led to movements to create a conceptual framework to build a health education curriculum, funded by the 3M Corporation (Sliepcevich, 1982). Although this curriculum was developed, by the 1970s it was clear that the curriculum was not being implemented in most districts (Cortese, 1993).

To try to improve the adoption of these curricula, the newly created U.S. Department of Education established an Office of Comprehensive School Health in 1978. It has since been eliminated. The Bureau of Health Education at the Centers for Disease Control and Prevention (CDC) was also established. This group has supported development of an elementary grades' health education curriculum known today as "Growing Healthy." CDC has also supported development of a comprehensive high school curriculum entitled "Teenage Health Teaching Modules" (Cortese, 1993). In addition to curriculum development, CDC has provided fiscal and technical assistance to school districts and to statewide efforts in the area of school health. Health education is the responsibility of several administrative agencies within the federal government. CDC is part of the Department of Health and Human Services, but many of the other responsibilities for school issues are located within the Department of Education. In 1994, a joint statement was issued by the Secretaries of Education and Health and Human Services supporting school health education efforts.

In 1993, a workshop was held to develop a working definition of comprehensive school health education (Kolbe, 1993). The other goal of the workshop was to develop a plan to help to institutionalize comprehensive school health education programs in the United States. In the Year 2,000 health objectives, over 100 specific objectives were related to school-age children and youth. More specifically, in the school health education area, one objective was to increase to at least 75% the proportion of the nation's elementary and secondary schools that provided planned and sequential kindergarten through 12th-grade quality school health education (Lavin, 1993; McGinnis, 1993).

In 1995, the Institute of Medicine adopted a provisional definition of a comprehensive school health program (Allensworth, Wyche, Lawson, et al., 1995):

> A comprehensive school health program is an integrated set of planned, sequential, school-affiliated strategies, activities and services designed to promote the optimal physical, emotional, social and educational development of students. The program involves and is supportive of families and is determined by the local community based on community needs, resources, standards and requirements. (p. 4)

In the same year, the School Health Policies and Programs Study (SHPPS) was established to measure policies and programs at the state, district, school, and classroom levels across multiple components of school health programs. All states responded to the state-level data collection effort. About 90% of states and districts require schools to offer health education. Some states specify topics to be included.

The most common topics required are HIV prevention, alcohol or drug use prevention, tobacco use prevention, dietary behaviors and nutrition, and disease prevention and control. From two thirds to three quarters of all states require these topics (Collins et al., 1995). Over 90% of states and districts have a written curriculum and guidelines or framework for health education. Of the states with requirements, about two thirds monitor compliance with the requirements (Collins et al., 1995). Often, in elementary schools, the teaching of health education is the responsibility of regular classroom teachers, whereas about two thirds of states require health education certification for secondary school health education programs. Although school nurses may often be involved in school health advisory councils that discuss health education programs, they are much less frequently involved in the actual delivery of the health education programs in a classroom setting.

Many different groups, including government agencies, have developed specific recommendations and guidelines about both program content and personnel for programs in specific topical areas such as AIDS, lifelong healthy eating, or tobacco use and prevention (CDC, 1994, 1996). A number of specific school health curricula have become well established, and many districts have developed their own innovative programs as well. The following is a brief review of some of the specifics of these guidelines and some programs.

In the area of tobacco use, recommendations are that programs to prevent and control use of tobacco include school policies on tobacco use as well as specific instruction about the short- and long-term negative physiologic and social consequences of tobacco use. Specific tobacco use prevention education, though important in all grades, should be especially intensive in middle/junior high school. Training should be provided to teachers, and peer leaders can often be incorporated at older grades. Similarly, involvement of families can be helpful (CDC, 1994).

School programs focused on healthy eating need to provide basic information about nutrition, change food services provided within the school to encourage healthier eating habits, and include school staff and family. Because nutrition and eating habits are linked to celebrations at all ages as well as to daily activity within the home, family background and cultural variability must be considered. Nutrition education instruction needs to be linked to children's developmental level and cultural backgrounds (CDC, 1996). Material for young children can rely on simple advice and concepts, whereas high-schoolers need more detailed, scientifically oriented advice. At all levels, programs need to recognize that eating patterns vary by cultural groups and that there are many different ways to develop a healthy diet yet to respect individual preferences and lifestyles. Recently, some more specific programs in some districts have included prevention of eating disorders also (Neumark-Sztainer, 1996). Eating disorders such as anorexia and bulimia nervosa are now the third most common chronic illness among adolescent girls in the United States, and a focus on dieting is common among female teenagers, so nutritional education in the junior and high school age groups needs to include these issues.

Some states have developed well-known comprehensive efforts, such as the Healthy Kids, Healthy Nebraska program in Nebraska public schools, which includes health education, physical education, guidance counseling and psychological services, health services, a focus on school environment, and parent and community partnerships (Davis & Allensworth, 1994). Iowa has also developed a comprehensive plan. In the most comprehensive plans, instruction on more controversial topics such as HIV/AIDS and death and dying are initially discussed as part of community partnerships so that the parents are in agreement with the schools about the presentation of these topics. In 1991, Michigan developed the Michigan Model for Comprehensive School Health Education the outcome of efforts in the state over a number of years. A complete K through 8 curriculum was provided, and a broad constituency of parents, religious leaders, and representatives of many government agencies in the state, such as the departments of education, mental health, public health, and social services, the state police, and the offices of highway safety planning and substance abuse services, were included in the planning. This curriculum has spread to many other states (Cortese, 1993). Some programs have incorporated both an effort at overall health education and some more disease-specific program goals. As one example, the Child and Adolescent Trial for Adolescent Health (CATCH) included both a school-based intervention program to promote health-enhancing behaviors in elementary school children and a specific focus on cardiovascular outcomes.

CONCLUDING COMMENTS

School health nurses and school health education programs have been a part of public school activities in the United States for many decades. In a rapidly changing society, one in which immigration rates are up (although not as high as they were during the era in which school health nursing was created in the United States) and the family is changing, whether through divorce or the need for both parents to work outside the home to earn a living, schools may need to give students more than education and a setting in which to learn. In the 1990s, many schools have begun to discuss the need to provide more services to children as families become more complicated and have less time for activities together. Whereas schools in the past have focused on specific educational activities and making schools themselves a safe place free of communicable diseases, schools in the future may need to become more active in helping students to stay healthy so that they can learn while in school. One way to do this is by the development of more health care services within the school, the topic of much of the rest of this book. Before looking in more detail at health care services in schools today, Chapter 3 will review the health of children today, focusing mostly on the United States.

CHAPTER 3

HEALTH STATUS OF CHILDREN

Past and Present

The health status of children in the United States varies, but most children today experience few lasting or significant illnesses as compared to children in the past. For most children today, childhood is a period of excellent or good health and one in which few children suffer significant abnormalities (Coiro, Zill, & Bloom, 1994; Roberts, 1973). Moreover, for most conditions, the state of child health in the United States has improved steadily over the past decades, partially because of advances in immunization programs, more stringent safety regulations, and advances in biomedical technology. Although this does not mean that children are never sick (in fact, most children experience bouts of minor illnesses, ranging from colds and minor fevers that do not even require medical attention to the potentially serious if untreated sore throats and ear infections), it does mean that the illnesses they experience are minor and transitory in nature, having no lasting impact on their ability to enjoy their childhood, attend school on a regular basis, and grow up into adulthood.

Although this is true for the majority of children, those who are not healthy bear a disproportionate burden of illness, and this burden tends to be concentrated most heavily in children from low-income families (Newacheck, Jameson, & Halfon, 1994). Given the relationships between income and minority group status in the United States, these children with greater health burdens are more often from minority groups, but the linkages are not simple or identical across all minority groups. In a recent national study, children's overall health rating was positively associated with higher levels of parental education, greater family income, and older maternal age at first birth (Coiro et al., 1994). Also, for children with chronic illnesses, an enjoyable childhood with regular school attendance becomes very difficult to achieve. Children with special problems due to their health status or familial and economic situation can be viewed a population that is more vulnerable or at risk in this society (Aday, 1993; Sherman, 1994). Recent discussions of children and problems have often focused on the concept of vulnerable children or children at risk, and it is helpful to examine both overall child health status data and more specialized data for vulnerable children.

This chapter will review the overall picture of health in children by examining the health of children across the major different age categories of childhood. It will also examine the health status of children who are more vulnerable, whether because of specific health problems or because of their social circumstances. Last, the chapter will link health status in children to the use of health care services and to other familial issues.

CURRENT OVERALL HEALTH

Overall health is always difficult to measure. Even the impact of illness can be conceptualized in several different ways. Epidemiologists describe the impact of disease in terms of "the five Ds": death, disease, disability, discomfort, and dissatisfaction (Haggerty, 1983; Patrick and Ellison, 1979). With children, as with adults, the best data are available for causes of death and the least for dissatisfaction level. Deaths are routinely registered by death certificates. Morbidity (sickness, disease) is routinely reported for only a few chronic conditions. Most morbidity data are gathered from special surveys, the largest of which is the National Health Interview (NHI) survey, a continuous nationwide household interview survey conducted by the National Center for Health Statistics (Massey, 1989). In 1988, a special survey that is one of the major current sources of information on child health in the United States included information on family patterns, child care, residential mobility, prenatal care, injuries, chronic conditions, and preventive health habits (Coiro et al., 1994). The next section of this chapter will look at the various stages of infancy and childhood and major health issues at each stage, using various sources of data, including the special child health survey. This section presents some overall data on morbidity and causes of mortality as a prelude to a more detailed examination of issues of child health in specific age categories.

One recent analysis of the special NHI survey data on child health explored the prevalence and impact of multiple childhood illnesses (Newacheck & Stoddard, 1994). This analysis included over 17,000 children under the age of 18 in United States households. Previous estimates of the percentage of children with chronic conditions have ranged from less than 5% to 30% (Newacheck & Taylor, 1992; Pless & Roghman, 1971; Starfield, 1991). One recent study, using data from before NHI special child health survey, reported that for children with chronic illnesses who were noninstitutionalized, 21% had two chronic conditions and 9% had three or more such conditions (Newacheck & Taylor, 1992). By the newer data, an estimated 19% of children younger than 18 years(about 12 million children nationwide) were reported to have one or more chronic conditions (Newacheck & Stoddard, 1994). This estimate included a comprehensive estimation of chronic illnesses, counting those that did not result in restriction of activity or a need for medical care as well as more serious illnesses. It was estimated that fewer than 5% of children had multiple (two or more) chronic conditions and that less than 1% of children had three or more such conditions (Newacheck & Stoddard, 1994). Respiratory conditions including hay fever, asthma, and other respiratory ailments, were the most commonly reported chronic problem. Other common chronic problems were digestive allergies, eczema, and skin allergies. For children with multiple problems, the top 10 pairs all included an allergy-related problem. Adolescents (11 to 17 years of age) were twice as likely as preschool children (birth to 6 years of age) to have multiple conditions. Boys were at greater risk than girls, and white children were more than twice as likely as African American children to report multiple chronic conditions. Though few children had multiple chronic conditions, they reported much greater morbidity across a number of measures, such as developmental delays, learning problems, days in bed, school absences, and activity limitation. They also used substantially more health care services than other children. Thus, morbidity data indicate the importance of chronic conditions and the presence of a positive health status for most children. But for children with chronic health problems, those with multiple illnesses have increased morbidity and health care use across many different measures.

Just as respiratory problems are the most commonly reported type of chronic illness for children, respiratory illnesses are the most frequent cause of restricted activity days for schoolchildren, followed by injuries and other infectious diseases (Pickett & Hanlon, 1990). Problems of growing importance for children, and very much linked to school issues and success in school, are emotional and behavioral problems. Accurate estimates of these problems are even more difficult to obtain than those for more common physical illnesses, but a report prepared by the Institute of Medicine (1989) estimated that at least 12% of children have a diagnosable mental illness. The percentage of children with learning disorders or diagnoses such as attention-deficit hyperactivity disorder (ADHD) is much larger and also creates major challenges for parents and for teachers in school settings.

Some limited data on leading causes of death in various age groups will provide a useful snapshot of the state of child health as reflected in mortality statistics. Although chronic conditions and injuries are now the major causes of death for children, patterns of child diseases and major health concerns are not the same from birth through the teenage years, and the importance of many chronic illnesses shows up more as children grow. Table 3.1 provides an introductory examination of the leading causes of death in major age groups. For the critical first year of life, perinatal conditions are the major cause. These include intrauterine growth problems, low birth weight, respiratory distress syndrome, and newborn problems due to complications of the pregnancy or complications of the placenta, cord, or membranes. After perinatal conditions, congenital anomalies and sudden infant death syndrome are the second and third major causes of death in those under 1 year of age. Most of these are causes of death that do not reappear in the other age groups, as compared to accidents and adverse events, which are important in other age groups of childhood (generally called injuries in those age groups). For children from ages 1 to 4, injuries are first, followed by congenital anomalies and malignant neoplasms. Though injuries remain the major cause of death in all the remaining child age groups (5-9, 10-14, and 15-24 years of age), the second and third causes vary in the different age groups. For those aged 5 to 9, malignant neoplasms are second (as they are for those from aged 10 to 14), followed by congenital anomalies for those aged 5 to 9 and malignant neoplasms for those aged 10 to 14. For the oldest group that includes children (15-24 years of age), injuries are first, followed by homicide and suicide. Though perinatal injuries and congenital anomalies are important, causes linked to the behavior of individuals, such as injuries, homicide, and suicide, become more important as children become older. The importance of these types of factors is making attention to behavioral and social aspects of child health more important than ever. Also, the important health care problems from morbidity statistics (such as respiratory illnesses) do not show up as major causes of death in children. This discrepancy illustrates the importance of examining both morbidity and mortality data to obtain a true picture of child health. Unlike old age, in which the health care problems from which people suffer become the diseases from which they die, childhood as a stage of life presents a more complicated health picture. Serious diseases from which children die are very uncommon, and are not the major health problems even among children with chronic health care conditions. To develop policy to deal with child health concerns, researchers and policy analysts need to focus both on common health problems, serious but nonfatal health problems, and diseases and factors such as injuries and suicides that lead to death in children.

Outcomes of Pregnancy: Maternal and Infant Health

Most experts agree that no period is more important to the good health of children than the months before birth, or the prenatal period. As a recent report from the Center for the Future of Children (1992) stated, "Children's health status begins with the conditions from which children emerge" (p. 7). The prenatal period can be the beginning of good health or the beginning of a lifetime of illness and shortened life expectancy. The death rate in this age group (about 1% of those born) is not exceeded in any age range until about age 65. Although the United States prides itself on having an outstanding health care system and being a healthy nation, this death rates places it behind most western European countries and many Asian ones also. As compared to earlier periods, most of this infant loss is due to factors that occur before and during pregnancy and delivery and result in death early in infancy, traditionally defined as the first month of life or neonatal period.

TABLE 3.1 Leading Causes of Death by Selected Age Groups of Children

Rank	Cause
Under 1 year	
1	Perinatal conditions
2	Congenital anomalies
3	Sudden infant death syndrome
4	Infections
5	Accidents and adverse events
1-4 years	
1	Injuries
2	Congenital anomalies
3	Malignant neoplasms
4	Homicides and legal interventions
5	Diseases of the heart
5-9 years	
1	Injuries
2	Malignant neoplasms
3	Congenital anomalies
4	Homicide
5	Diseases of the heart
10-14 years	
1	Injuries
2	Malignant neoplasms
3	Suicide
4	Homicide
5	Congenital anomalies
15-24 years	
1	Injuries
2	Homicide
3	Suicide
4	Malignant neoplasms
5	Diseases of the heart

SOURCE: Adapted from Monthly Vital Statistics Report, 42 (11), 1994 from the National Center for Health Statistics.

The single greatest hazard to the health of infants is low birth weight (less than 2,500 g), which occurs in about 7% of all live births (U.S. Department of Health and Human Services [USDHHS], 1991). Almost three quarters of deaths in the first month and 60% of all infant deaths occur among low-birth-weight babies. As compared to congenital malformations, another major cause of death in the first 30 days of life but one that is often present before prenatal care begins, low birth weight generally reflects second- and third-trimester events and thus is linked to several preventable risks (McCormick & Brooks-Gunn, 1989; USDHHS, 1991). For low birth weight, lack of prenatal care is one preventable factor, along with maternal smoking, use of alcohol and other drugs, and pregnancy before age 18. Low birth weight is linked to both race and income. African American infants are twice as likely as white infants to be of low birth weight. Low income and low educational levels are also linked to small babies.

Although low birth weight's contribution to morbidity is less well established than it's contribution to mortality, evidence does exist that links low birth weight to neurodevelopmental handicaps and even to the development of other illnesses that require hospitalization in the first year of life (McCormick, 1987). Many of these problems and developmental delays appear to decrease over time, so except for the smallest low-birth-weight babies, longer term health is good if the baby survives the first critical year of life.

In the NHI Survey of parents of children, when parents were asked to rate the child's health, 42% of those with a low-birth-weight baby rated the child's health as excellent with no limiting conditions, versus 58% of those with a non-low-birth-weight baby (Coiro et al., 1994). In the same study, 62% of parents of children with no chronic health care problem rated the baby's health as excellent versus only 40% of parents whose children had one or more chronic health problems. Developmental delays for these infants under 1 year of age were strongly related to child's birth weight and, to a lesser extent, to presence of chronic conditions. Only 2% of non-low-birth-weight babies experienced developmental delays, versus 11% of low-birth-weight babies in the 1,500-g to 2,500-g category and versus over 30% of babies who survived and who initially weighed less than 1,500 g. For infants with a chronic condition, almost 7% were reported by parents as having a developmental delay in the first year of life, versus only 1% of those without a chronic condition.

One of the major ways to improve the health of children in this age group is to improve prenatal health care and, to a lesser extent, to improve neonatal intensive care. Discrepancies exist in the United States between different ethnic and economic groups in the receipt of prenatal care. Eliminating these differentials would improve the health of infants. Recent policy reviews have emphasized the need to focus on poor families and women with high-risk pregnancies (Raccine, Joyce, & Grossman, 1992).

Younger Children

Once past the first year of life, injuries and infectious conditions become the most important impediments to health for preschool children. Infectious diseases of the past, such as pneumonia and influenza, which in 1950 accounted for about 25% of deaths in children from ages 1 through 5, now account for only 10% of deaths (Perrin, Guyer, & Lawrence, 1992). The receipt of appropriate immunizations in this age group is critical, for preventing both immediate and longer term health care problems. In addition to the well-known vaccinations for the once-common childhood illnesses of measles, mumps, and rubella, there are vaccinations for the once lethal problems of pertussis and polio. Newer vaccines are becoming available for such problems as chicken pox, a minor problem if one considers mortality but nevertheless an important vaccination for reduction of morbidity in children and lost work time for parents.

New problems such as injuries, environmental toxins, family violence, and developmental disorders are now more important health problems in this age group. Homicide linked to child abuse, for example, is now one of the five major causes of death in children from 1 through 4 years of age, although only in a small number of families. More commonly, this is the age of injuries due to household hazards and falls. Head injuries as well as other bodily injuries from falls increase, and injuries due to poisons and water (both drownings and scalds from hot water) become important health threats. Whereas injuries are the most common cause of death in this age group, upper respiratory illnesses are the most common cause of illness (Haggerty, 1983). Common types of respiratory problems are the common cold, sore throats, laryngitis, and otitis media (ear infections). The treatment of otitis media has become more controversial, with debate over the appropriate role of antibiotics and of surgical intervention in the form of tubes to open the ear canals. Less common are lower-respiratory infections such as bronchitis and pneumonia. Most respiratory infections in this age group are caused by viruses and will have a positive outcome even without medical intervention. Some estimates are that children acquire hundreds of viral infections by the age of 10 to 12. Though only a minority of the total respiratory infections in this age group are bacterial, they include some of the most important streptococcal infections, some otitis media, and some forms of meningitis. Bacterial infections are treated very effectively by antibiotics and, if untreated, have serious outcomes for children. A major role of clinical medicine in this age group (and thus the importance of adequate access to care) is to differentiate between bacterial and viral illnesses.

Social factors are important in differentiating between children in poor health or with limiting conditions. In the NHI survey data, the percentage of children reported to be in fair to poor health is highest (11.6%) in the lowest income category of less than $10,000 a year of family income, both for children from 1 to 2 years of age and for those from 3 to 4 years of age (Coiro et al., 1994). In the next two income categories of $10,000 to 420,000 and $20,000 to $35,000 a year, about 4% of 1- to 2-year olds and 5.5% of 3- to 4-year-olds are in fair to poor health. For those aged 3 to 4 years, the percentage decreases further to about 2.5% in the two highest income categories of $35,000 to $50,000 a year and over $50,000. For children aged 1 to 2, the percentage decreases to about 3% and then increases a bit in the highest income category back to almost 5%. For education, the patterns are more consistent, with almost 12% of children aged 1 to 2 whose parents have less than a high school education being in fair to poor health versus only 1% of those whose parents have some graduate education. For those 3 to 4 years of age, the pattern is the same, with percentages decreasing from almost 8% to about 3%. At the other end of the health spectrum, trends are similar for both income and education. For example, 40% of the 1- to 4-year-old children in the lowest income category are in excellent health with no limiting conditions versus about 65% in the highest income category.

School-Age Children

Many aspects of health for school-age children are similar to those for the 1- to 4-year-old group. Unintentional injuries and infectious illnesses are the major reasons that children in this age group miss school. The major sources of hospitalization for children are respiratory problems, injuries, gastrointestinal problems, nervous system and sense organ problems, infections, and congenital anomalies. Injuries jump out as an important factor in mortality, hospitalization, and overall morbidity. The specific types of injuries do change as children enter school. Injuries within the home and from scalds, burns, and water decline, and as children grow older, playground and sports injuries become more common, although motor vehicle injuries account for the largest proportion of mortality linked to unintentional injury in this age group. Sadly, homicide is one of the five leading causes of death for school-age children, often linked to child abuse. It is the only leading cause of death for children in this age group that has been increasing over the past 30 years (McCormick & Gunn, 1989). Most childhood homicides are perpetrated by parents and other relatives. Injuries are now the major cause of childhood mortality, morbidity, and disability (Guyers & Eller, 1990; Perrin et al., 1992; Starfield, 1991).

The longer term consequences of early, serious child health problems in infancy and the preschool period are under debate. One major research question has been the extent to which early child health problems affect parental perception of child health later on in childhood. Literature on younger children describes the "vulnerable child syndrome," or a situation in which a child has a relatively severe health problem in infancy that by early childhood leads to a sense of special vulnerability and greater protectiveness by the parents (Green & Solnit, 1964; Levy, 1980). A study was conducted with 1,877 children between the ages of 8 to 10 years in 13 different sites in the United States (McCormick, Brooks-Gunn, Workman-Daniels, & Peckham, 1993). Parental rating of current child health and resistance or susceptibility to health problems was not related to events in infancy, including low birth weight. The personal rating was linked to current child health problems. These results reinforce the validity of maternal assessment of child health and confirm that low birth weight in and of itself does not necessarily affect the health of the child or perceptions of that child's health by the time school is begun (McCormick et al., 1993).

Many of the same infectious diseases found in preschool children are common in school-age children, but the amount of otitis media declines as children grow. Minor infectious illnesses and minor injuries are common, with most children experiencing from four to six episodes a year. Most of these episodes are minor and often result in little if any restriction of normal activities. Many over-the-counter medications and remedies are purchased for these problems. One respiratory problem whose incidence is increasing in recent years is asthma, especially among children living in cities, possibly as a result of environmental exposures (USDHHS, 1991). This problem can be more serious, especially if not treated by medical personnel. Recent studies have estimated the prevalence may be as high as 6% to 7% (Gergen, Mullally, & Evans, 1988). Even for less serious respiratory problems than asthma, evidence is available that access to and early contact with medical services are associated with a reduction of length of illness, severity of symptoms, and progression to more severe stages of illness that may result in hospitalization (Hadley, 1982; McCormick & Brooks-Gunn, 1989; Perrin et al., 1992; Starfield, 1985). Because easy access to health services for minor problems is important, issues about access to health care at schools becomes an issue for this age group. Not all parents have health insurance or a regular source of care, and even for those that do, the growth of two-income households makes it more difficult for parents to have children seen by health care personnel for these common, minor illnesses.

If children receive a physical examination, different major health problems are discovered than through the examination of mortality or morbidity data. In order of frequency, the most common problems noted through a physical examination are dental problems, skin pathology, ear problems, eye problems, neuromuscular/joint problems, and cardiovascular problems (Starfield, 1991). Different sources of information indicate different types of child health problems. In a comparison of literature reviews, household surveys, and 6-year data from health maintenance organization (HMO) records, asthma, visual impairments, and hearing impairments were the three most prevalent problems in the literature reviews, and visual impairments, allergies, and asthma were the most prevalent in the household survey and the HMO data, but allergies ranked first in the HMO data, whereas visual impairments ranked first in the survey (Starfield, 1991).

As children begin school, issues of emotional and behavioral health and learning disorders become much more important. Learning disorders often do not appear until a child is enrolled in a school setting, and many other behavioral health problems also first are recognized in that setting. One problem that was not diagnostically identified among school-age children in previous generations is ADHD, or problems with attention and information processing (Levine, 1982). Several recent studies have identified a set of problems as the "new morbidities" of childhood and have listed behavior disorders as the most common of these, along with lead poisoning, child abuse, and developmental delay (Newacheck & Starfield, 1988; Perrin et al., 1992). Although experts disagree on the diagnosis and treatment of these problems, in many school settings they have become a major health problem for which children receive medication during the school day, along with asthma that requires the use of inhalers. Studies estimate that between five and 20% of all children in school may have some combination of learning problems and behavioral disorders (Butler, Rosenbaum & Palfrey, 1987; Levine & Satz, 1984; McCormick & Brooks-Gunn, 1989; Perrin et al., 1992). These issues will be discussed in more detail in a later section.

Data from the NHI special survey on child health provide more information about children from 5 through 11 years of age, roughly the age of children discussed in this section. As with younger children, worse health status is linked to socioeconomic indicators such as income and education of the parents. Fourteen percent of children in families with the lowest income (less than $10,000) are in fair or poor health as compared to only 6% of those in families earning $50,000 or more a year (Coiro et al., 1994). The pattern is similar, but the differentials smaller, for education. One other important finding linked to the issue of school health programs discussed in later chapters of this book concerns the presence of a regular source of care and of health insurance. For all children from ages 5 through 11, 14% do not have any health insurance, and 9% have no regular source for routine medical care. Children from Hispanic-origin families are much more likely to have no health insurance (27% do not) compared to only 11% of children from non-Hispanic families. For lack of a regular source of care, the comparisons are 16% versus about 8%. Children in families in which the parents are not high school graduates are much more likely to have no health insurance (27%) than those whose parents are college graduates (7.5%) or those whose parents have some graduate school (5.5%). Children with family income in the lowest two categories (under $20,000 income) are more likely to have no health insurance (about 25% in both groups, compared to only 6% in the two highest income categories of $35,000 a year or more). Similar trends hold for lack of a regular source of care. The two lowest income groups have almost triple the percentage of children without a regular source of care in the two highest income groups, roughly 15% versus 5%. With education, the differential is over fourfold, with only 5% of children in families with college graduates or higher having no regular source of care versus almost 20% of those whose parents do not have a high school diploma. These figures help to illustrate the important role that the availability of more health care services in schools could play in improving the health of children, especially children from families with lower levels of income and education.

Adolescents

Many of the same factors that affect children in elementary school, such as minor infectious diseases and behavioral and environmental problems, also affect adolescents. In adolescence, however, several critical differences begin. One of these is that responsibility for health and health behavior increasingly shifts from the parent to the teenager. Another is that many more areas of activity with health consequences become choices for adolescents: whether to engage in risky and unhealthy behaviors such as smoking or drinking; whether to engage in sexual intercourse and, if one does, whether to use protection from unwanted pregnancies; and whether to drive and how careful one is about driving situations, such as being sure to wear seatbelts, not driving under the influence of alcohol, and not driving with large numbers of other teens in the car so that the driver loses concentration or becomes susceptible to pressures of driving too fast.

Adolescence is not a clearly defined period of years. Some health sources present data for those aged 10 through 19, whereas others call ages 10 through 24 the years of adolescence and young adulthood and present data separately for those aged 10 through 14 and those aged 15 through 24 as in Table 2-1, which show causes of mortality by age group. Still others define ages 12 through 17 years as adolescence. Almost all sources include the teenage years during which a child is still in secondary school, or the period from 7th grade through 12th grade. This section will present data from a number of different sources, so the exact age group covered will vary somewhat.

Because adolescence is often a period of low use of medical care, it was once assumed that teens were healthier than younger age groups of children. Increasingly, this does not seem to be accurate, but adolescents are reluctant to use medical care, especially the physicians that parents use, and this may have contributed to the idea that teenagers are healthier than other age groups (Haggerty, 1983; Perrin et al., 1992). On the basis of mortality measures, adolescents 10 through 19 years of age represent the only segment of the U.S. population in which mortality rates have not declined rapidly during the past 20 years (Fingerhut & Kleinman, 1989).

Motor vehicle crash injuries, suicide, and homicide and other violence-related causes are the major causes of mortality in adolescence. All of these are linked to behavior. Many are linked to risk-taking behaviors and poor health habits. Others relate to unhealthy social environments and excessive concern about problems at school, at home, or with maturation.

Unintentional injures account for half of all deaths among people ages 15 through 24, with three quarters of these deaths involving motor vehicles. Over half of all fatal motor vehicle crashes in this age group involve alcohol. Speeding is also more often a factor in teen traffic injuries than in adult injuries. In addition, teens use seatbelts less often than do adults (McCormick & Brooks-Gunn, 1989; USDHHS, 1991). In one study, nearly 60% of 8th and 10th graders reported not using seatbelts on their most recent ride in an automobile (USDHHS, 1991). These data illustrate one of the dilemmas of working with adolescents and trying to convince them to adopt healthy behaviors. This is a period of life in which people feel invincible and invulnerable to many of the negatives outcomes of their behavior, discounting the possibility of risk (Irwin & Millstein, 1986). Youth do not easily respond to the threat of developing a serious illness 30 years later. They do not even respond to more immediate threats of serious injury and disability. Convincing children in this period to refrain from risky behaviors is a difficult challenge.

The adolescent years are a time of changing health habits and experimentation with many things. It is during this period that health habits are formed that are most likely to persist into adulthood and even into the later years of life. Helping adolescents to make better choices is one of the most important roles of health care providers for people in this age group. The dominant preventable health problems of adolescents are injuries and violence (USDHHS, 1991). Seventy-three percent of the deaths that occur between the ages of 10 and 19 are attributable to intentional and unintentional injuries and violence (Perrin et al., 1992). Homicide is the second leading cause of death among all adolescents and is the number one cause among African American youth (USDHHS, 1991). Racial differences in homicide rates are diminished greatly when socioeconomic factors are taken into account, so homicide is of greatest risk to poor youth who may live in communities in which violence is viewed as an acceptable part of life and a way to resolve differences. As with automobile injuries, use of alcohol is often linked to homicides.

Suicide is one of the major causes of death, especially for young white men. Over the last 30 years, the death rate from suicide among white males has tripled. White females attempt suicide at rates higher than African American females but tend not to die from the attempts at as high a rate as do males, partially because women often are found and saved from such methods as overdoses of pills, whereas men more often employ guns and hanging as methods of suicide.

Adolescents now are likely to adopt what were previously "adult" behaviors at earlier ages. Substance abuse of many types often begins in adolescence. Use of alcohol is a major health problem, with some studies reporting that as many 93% of high school seniors have had a drink in the last month. Even if these figures are exaggerated due to self-reports by teens, evidence is strong that more than one of out every three high school seniors have had five or more drinks in a row in any 2-week period, a measure of serious abuse of alcohol versus fleeting exposure (Johnston, Bachman, & O'Malley, 1984; Starfield, 1991). Alcohol use is important not only as its own risk but because of its association with motor vehicle crashes and violence. Some studies report use of alcohol at ever-younger ages, such as 28% of eighth graders reporting occasions of heavy drinking (USDHHS, 1991). Among young people from ages 18 to 24, drinking is more prevalent than in any other age group. College campuses have recently increased attention to drinking as a problem, and many campuses ban alcohol from most events.

Alcohol is a legal substance in the society, although illegal for youths under 21. Use of illegal drugs besides alcohol has been declining in the United States among young people who remain in school, but experimentation often begins as early as the eighth grade. Causing this activity to be viewed more negatively by students has been one of the foci of drug education programs, both in the schools and with general media advertisements. Recent estimates are that about 3% of high school seniors may be heavy users of cocaine (Starfield, 1991).

Smoking as a negative health habit is receiving great amounts of attention currently. The earlier cigarette smoking begins, the less likely a smoker is to quit. Of high school seniors who smoke, three fourths report smoking a first cigarette as young as Grade 9. Although rates of teen smoking among boys have been declining, smoking among girls has not. Beyond cigarette use, snuff and chewing tobacco are used, especially among boys. Although this health problem is not as linked to violence as alcohol and drug use are, it is strongly linked to the development of chronic health problems in later adult life. As recent releases of information from tobacco companies have made clear, marketing efforts targeted at teenagers have been one approach to "hook" this age group to the use of tobacco. Many of these approaches (cartoon characters such as Joe Camel and use of merchandise coupons so that students wear clothing that advertises tobacco) are now illegal, or companies have stated they will no longer fund these efforts. However, one current growth trend in tobacco use is use of cigars. Though much of the social appeal seems aimed at more affluent groups than teenagers, especially young professionals in their 20s and beyond, the trend may extend to teenagers as it grows.

Goals for adolescent health have to focus on development of healthy habits, control of unhealthy substances, and development of appropriate attitudes toward sexuality. Sexuality-related issues include the prevention of unwanted teenage pregnancy and the control of the spread of sexually transmitted diseases, including HIV infection. Estimates are that over three quarters of adolescents have engaged in sexual intercourse by age 19, making education in this area critical. Issues of education around sexual topics are often among the most controversial for school systems. Some experts have suggested that health care providers would be good sources of this type of information. But in reality, discussions about sexuality and related topics are most easily addressed in schools or in the home because adolescents between the ages of 10 and 18 make limited visits to health care providers (1.6 visits a year, on average). This number is even lower among African American adolescents (0.9 visits) (Office of Technology Assessment, 1991). Providing services and education to adolescents is a challenge, and the role of schools in either education or service provision becomes particularly controversial if teens are involved and if sexuality is addressed as a topic.

The NHI survey data set did include children up through the age of 17. Teenagers from ages 12 to 17 had the highest proportion with what has been called the "new morbidity of childhood": learning problems and emotional and behavioral problems. Almost 25% of adolescents were reported by their parents to have a developmental delay, learning disability, or emotional or behavioral problem. The percentage of boys with these problems is larger than the percentage of girls (29% versus 21% for those from 12 to 17 years of age). Higher proportions of white children than African American children were reported to have these problems, and there were no differences between Hispanics and non-Hispanics (Coiro et al., 1994). Previous data indicate that lower-income children are at higher risk of psychological disorders, and such children are over represented in special education, making these findings surprising. One interpretation is that African American and Hispanic families interviewed in the survey were under reporting these problems due to unfamiliarity with wording used, as well as due to less willingness to seek mental health services or admit the use of such services (Zill & Schoenborn, 1990).

Recently, researchers have developed new measures of adolescent health status to try to account for the complex factors included in health at this stage of life (Starfield et al., 1993, 1995). This new instrument, called the Child Health and Illness Profile-Adolescent Edition (CHIP-AE), covers aspects of health in six domains: discomfort, satisfaction with health, disorders, achievement of social expectations, risks, and resilience. Acutely ill teenagers report more physical discomfort, more minor illnesses, and lower physical fitness. Chronically ill teenagers report more activity limitations, more long-term medical disorders, more dissatisfaction with their health, and less physical fitness than other teenagers in the sample (Starfield et al., 1996). The fact that age, sex and socioeconomic status were not the major explanations for the effects of illness on health demonstrates the usefulness of this approach for future research. One other advantage of this new approach for collecting information on adolescent health is that it relies on answers from the teenagers themselves rather than their parents.

LINKAGES WITH POVERTY AND MINORITY STATUS

Although linkages between child health and poverty have already been discussed briefly, this topic is very important to a discussion of expanded roles for school health programs, including the provision of services within a school setting. Thus, a more comprehensive review of findings in this area is useful. Poverty negatively influences child health and development along a number of dimensions (Aber et al., 1997; Krieger, Rowley, Herman, Avery, & Phillips,1993; Moffitt, 1997; Newacheck et al., 1994; Nickens, 1995). Given the relationships in American society today between poverty and minority/racial/ethnic status, any discussion of the impact of poverty on health also raises issues of linkages by race/ethnicity (Krieger et al., 1993).

Data On Linkages Between Poverty, Education and Health

Children's overall health ratings are strongly associated with a variety of socioeconomic measures in most studies, including parental education, family income, and maternal age at first birth. In the NHI survey of children, whereas 68% of children whose parents had some graduate school education were rated favorably on their health, only 35% of children whose parents had less than a high school education were (Coiro et al., 1994). For income in the same data set, the range was from 64% in upper income families to 35% in low-income families. In a recent government publication that reviewed data from the NHI survey in 1988, 1989, and 1990, children under age 18 living in families with annual incomes under $10,000 reported a higher percentage who were limited in activity, a higher percentage with fair or poor health status, and a higher percentage with a hospitalization in the last 12 months than did children in households with higher incomes (National Center for Health Statistics, 1996). In the same data sets, children under 18 years of age had higher rates of hospitalization in families in which the responsible adult member had less than 12 years of education than in families where the responsible adult was better educated.

A recent review of data from the National Health Examination Survey and the National Health and Nutrition Examination Survey (surveys in which physicians examine children and conduct laboratory tests, removing the role of the parent as an intermediary in data collection that occurs in many other surveys about health of children) found worse health for poor children on many of the measures, including measures of problems such as dental health and vision that are not often discussed in surveys whose methods focus on reports from the parents (Newacheck et al., 1994). For most measures of dental health, poor children had more oral debris, more decayed and missing teeth, and more periodontal disease. Only for occlusion of the teeth was the relationship weak. Youth from low-income families had 50% more non-acne-related skin conditions. For visual health, youths from poor families actually had better unaided visual acuity than did youths from high-income families. Once eyeglasses use was considered, however, the relationship was reversed, with low-income youths less likely to have adequate refraction. Tests for hearing were included as part of the medical examinations. Abnormalities of the eardrum due to infection, allergy or other medical conditions are a sign of middle-ear disease and are correlated with decreased hearing capacity. Low-income youth were significantly more likely to have eardrum abnormalities, an indication of present or past middle-ear disease (Newacheck et al., 1994). Problems with dental disease, uncorrected vision, and untreated ear infections are among the most common concerns of nurses and others who work in schools with low-income children. Poor vision and hearing often lead to immediate problems of success in school. Both lack of health insurance and the subsequent funds to pay for these health services and lack of ability to take children to the services if the funds to pay for them are available are major concerns of school health personnel.

Health interview survey data support the results of these examination data. In 1992, poor children scored lower on all measures of limitation of activity due to poor health, including bed days, school-loss days, and limitation of activity. Longer term relationships between activity levels also varied by family income. The proportion of children and youth in families with incomes below $10,000 who were limited in their activities due to chronic illness was twice as high as for children from families earning $35,000 annually or more (Newacheck et al., 1994). Findings for behavioral health problems show a similar pattern of relationships. Children and youth from families with lower incomes scored higher than those from higher income families on six behavioral problem subscales: antisocial behavior, anxiety and depression, headstrong behavior, hyperactivity, immaturity and dependence, and conflict and withdrawal. The largest income-related difference was found for the antisocial behavior (cheats or lies, bullies, is cruel or mean, disobedient in school, not sorry after misbehaving, trouble getting along with others, and destructive).

Poverty and Ethnic/Minority Status

Linking these type of findings to issues about minority health becomes more complicated. For years, minority health in the United States was considered a unitary phenomenon, with all minority groups considered in comparison to whites (Nickens, 1995). Many times, although minorities were discussed, the actual data were available only for African Americans versus whites. But in the late 1990s, the United States is an increasingly multiethnic society. Whereas in 1980, non-Hispanic whites were about 80% of the U.S. population, by 1990 they were only 75% of the total population, and the figure is expected to be even lower by the year 2000 census. The most rapidly growing part of the U.S. population is minority groups, and the census projects that by the year 2050, the United States will be half minority (Bureau of the Census, 1992). Hispanics are increasing more rapidly than any other minority group. Moreover, among non-Hispanic whites and African Americans (the only two groups for whom studies are available), the class gradient in mortality rates overall is increasing. Poor whites have higher mortality in relation to high income whites than in the past, and poor African Americans have higher mortality rates in relation to high-income African Americans than in the past (Pappas, Morris, & Smith et al., 1982).

One line of research that has particularly focused on interactions between racial/ethnic status and poverty is research about infant mortality rates. As was mentioned in the section on health of infants, infant mortality rates in the United States are higher in the aggregate among poor and less educated women, and African American-to-white differentials in infant mortality have been substantial for decades and increasing in recent years, with a differential as high as 2.4 (Krieger et al., 1993; Nickens, 1995). To complicate matters, African American women appear to have problematic birth outcomes regardless of their socioeconomic position, so that they fare worse than white women at every economic level, with the economic disadvantage continuing somewhat even among highly educated African American women (Collins and David, 1990; Krieger et al., 1993; Schoendorft, Hogue, Kleinman, & Rowley, 1992). Another factor that complicates understanding the relationship between racial/ethnic status and poverty as regards studies of health outcomes is that Hispanic health data, especially on infant mortality, show better health outcomes even though the Hispanic population has rates of poverty similar to those of the African American population. Although often labeled the "Hispanic paradox," this finding should more accurately be labeled the "Mexican American paradox" because it involves birth outcomes among Mexican American and Mexican-born women (Beccera, Hogue, Atrash, & Perez, 1991; Markides & Coreil, 1986; Nevolo, Wise, & Kleinman, 1991). Despite comparable sociodemographic factors, low-birth-weight rates and infant mortality rates among Mexican American and Mexican-born women in the United States are lower than among African American women at every economic level and at all levels combined (Beccera et al., 1991). Although some experts argue that these results might be spurious and result from underascertainment of infant deaths among Mexican Americans, many other experts believe they represent a larger problem of a persistent inability to explain a myriad of racial/ethnic differences in health (Krierger et al., 1993). As new research is developed, important points to consider are inclusion of more consistent and better measures of both social class and racial/ethnic classifications, inclusion of contextual factors of neighborhoods in which people live, and inclusion of the impact of racism and discrimination on the lives (and thus the health) of individuals. In addition, better understanding of linkages between these factors and access to the health care delivery system is needed (Krieger et al., 1993; Nickens, 1995).

Teen Pregnancy as a Special Area of Linkage

One last area of importance in the relation of poverty and race/ethnicity to the health of children is the issue of teen pregnancy. This topic links the health of teenage girls who become pregnant with the health of the next generation of children. Teenage childbearing is associated with some undesirable outcomes for both the teenage mothers and their babies (Lewit, 1992). For the babies, rates of preterm birth are higher, as are rates of low birth weight and infant mortality. Even after infancy, the children of teenage mothers have more problems in school, score lower on IQ tests, and have more emotional problems. For the mothers, the negative effects are not so much on physical health status as on social development and changes. Teenage mothers are less likely to finish high school and college, and they earn lower incomes in later life, setting up a lifetime of concerns for these young women (Lewit, 1992; Miller, Fine, & Adams-Taylor, 1989). The birthrate for African American teens has been more than twice the birthrate for white teens in the 20-year period from 1970 to 1989 (Lewit, 1992). The birthrates for unmarried African American women, both teens and adults, were three to four times the birthrate for unmarried white teens and adults.

Special programs can help to improve the life chances of these young women and their babies. Changes in school policies over the last two decades that allow teen mothers to stay in school and that sometimes include the provision of child care in the school setting along with classes on child rearing are helpful. Preventing childbirths is also helpful. In both of these situations, on-site health care services in school settings may aid in prevention of teen births and improvement of both prenatal care and infant care. Two recent reports about special projects that included nurse home visits demonstrated that the program improved not just the infant care of the poor young mothers but also an array of social and health outcomes for as long as 15 years following the childbirth (Kitzman et al., 1997; Olds et al., 1997). As an editorial about the two programs and a new book based on one of the programs concluded, only a small portion of the negative outcomes of teen mothers and their children could have been prevented by delaying motherhood beyond the age of 20 years (Maynard, 1997; Moffitt, 1997). Most negative impacts came from the mother's own personal background, suggesting that the positive impact of many of the special programs is to help change the personal circumstances of the young mothers, including their health behaviors, child-rearing practices, and educational achievements. These findings link to the last section of this chapter, on relationships between access to and use of health care and family structures.

ACCESS TO AND USE OF HEALTH CARE

One of the major goals outlined in *Healthy People 2000* (USDHHS, 1994) was to achieve access to preventive services for all Americans. Given that overall health of American children is good, preventive services are especially important to child health and provide one of the ways to improve the overall health of children in the United States. Early and sustained use of health care is often critical in identifying, treating, and monitoring childhood conditions. Special federal data on the health of the nation's children included information on four different indicators of access to health care services: health insurance coverage, last visit, regular source of care, and regular provider at that source (Coiro et al., 1994).

About three quarters of children aged 0 to 17 were covered by private health insurance, with another 10% covered by Medicaid, leaving 14.5% with no form of health insurance.

Health insurance enhances access to both preventive care and routine sickness care. Most children do receive routine medical care; only 16% had not had such care at least once in the last 2 years. Younger children are more likely to receive routine care. Only 4% of infants had received no care in the past 2 years versus 22% of children from ages 2 through 17. Children in the South and the West were at a disadvantage in receipt of routine care, as were children living outside metropolitan areas. Ethnicity was also important. Native American children were twice as likely as other groups to lack health insurance, with 38% having no coverage. The rate of lack of health insurance was also twice as high for Hispanic children, with 27% having no health insurance versus only 13% of non-Hispanic children.

For the majority of children that had received routine medical care, respondents were asked if there was a particular clinic, health center, or doctor's office where the child usually received health care. About 10% of children had no usual place for routine care, up from 6% in a similar question in a 1980 survey (Coiro et al., 1994). A related question asked parents if there was a particular place where children received care when sick and if there was a particular person whom they saw at this place. Though only 7% of children did not receive sick care from a regular place, 19% did not receive care from a particular provider. Nonwhite children were less likely to have received care from a particular provider of sick care. Whereas only 16% of white children lacked such a provider, 32% of African American children and 44% of Native American children lacked such a provider. Hispanic children were also less likely to have such a provider. As with other types of data, we see linkages between limited access by minorities and by the poor. Children in the lowest income bracket were two to four times less likely than those in the highest income bracket to have medical insurance and a particular provider of care. They were also less likely to have had routine care in the last 2 years. Perhaps not surprisingly, given the availability of Medicaid to some of the poorest families and not to those in the next income category, similar proportions of children in the $10,000 to $20,000 income bracket and the lowest income bracket lacked access to health care.

The report also included some indicators of children's use of health care services (Coiro et al., 1994). Some information was collected on number of contacts the child had with health care providers, the number of days that an illness or injury kept the child in bed more than half the day (bed days), and the number of short-stay hospital visits. Younger children had more doctor visits, had more hospital episodes, and spent more days in bed than older children. Few differences were important by race/ethnicity or area of the country. Native Americans do report more hospital episodes than other racial/ethnic groups. This may be due to the lack of health insurance and thus the reliance upon the hospital to provide more care. Actual use of services was less related to parental socioeconomic status than were the measures of access to care already discussed, especially the number of doctor visits and number of bed days. Number of hospital episodes was related to measures of socioeconomic status, with disadvantaged children having much higher rates of hospitalization. These rates of use may reflect actual differences in severity of illness or injury. Children from lower-income families do have poorer health status overall and more developmental disorders than do other children. Thus, these data suggest the need for more access to both routine and sick care services for disadvantaged children. Because one service now provided in the United States to most children, whatever the parental levels of income is, school services, these findings reinforce an important potential role for schools in the provision of needed health care services to all children, but especially low-income children.

CHAPTER 4

MODELS OF SCHOOL HEALTH DELIVERY

The Growth of School-Based Clinics and Centers

This chapter will review the development of school-based clinics for health services for children in the United States. To understand the role of school-based clinics in the care of children, some understanding of existing models of organization of health care delivery systems in the United States is helpful, and that is the focus of the first portion of this chapter. The second portion focuses on models of school-based clinics and programs in various states.

DELIVERY OF HEALTH CARE IN THE UNITED STATES

Models both of delivering health care services and of dealing with health problems have been changing in the last 20 years. Traditionally, the model for delivery of health care services in the United States was the fee-for-service, individual or small practitioner model. In this model, people generally decided for themselves and their family from whom to obtain care and paid for that care at the time it was delivered. The growth of health insurance changed this model for major episodes of care that resulted in hospitalization but not for acute care services, which tended to remain on a fee-for-service basis, with the fee paid at the time the services were delivered. In hospital services, the typical model was that insured patients received a bill after the services were provided, and much of the bill was covered by insurance.

The 1950s have often been described as the "Golden Age of Medicine," in which the idealized image of an individual private practitioner giving care to a child as part of a family arose (Burnham, 1982). In truth, we know that this period was ideal only for middle-class and affluent families. However, there was a cultural expectation about ideal types of care (and for physicians, about ideal types of patients and practices) that was later reflected in such TV shows as *Marcus Welby, M.D.* which showed a grandfatherly physician dispensing medical care, sympathy, and counseling to a grateful child and family.

By the 1960s, many parts of the country began to see a growth of alternative delivery models for health care, including the prepaid group practice (PPGP), later renamed the health maintenance organization (HMO) in the Nixon era as an alternative delivery style for many working families, followed by the independent practice association (IPA). By 1965, an alternative payment approach for poor families became Medicaid, a joint federal-state program to pay for health care services for some categories of the poor, including many poor children, especially those in female-headed poor households. Previously, the urban poor had received care from county or municipal clinics or had depended on the good will of a local physician. Depending on the good will of local physicians had also been the major way the rural poor received care. Although the initial growth of Medicaid led to an increase in the ability of poor families to select private providers for their children, the efforts of states to hold down spending on Medicaid often led to a low fee structure. Both the low fee structure and transportation and language difficulties often led poor families to end up obtaining care from their more traditional sources of clinics and county health departments.

As managed care (PPGPs, HMOs, IPAs) has grown in the 1980s and 1990s, some states have begun to look to it as a better way to provide health care services to the Medicaid population. Arizona has been a leader in that effort. It has maintained a completely managed-care-model Medicaid program since the mid-1980s (before that time, Arizona was the only state not participating in Medicaid). Because the next chapter of this book focuses in more detail on school-based clinics within Arizona, it is important to consider the applicability to this newer model of care of models developed to make school clinics work in other states with more traditional Medicaid programs. It is especially important because many more states are now beginning to switch the emphasis of their Medicaid programs to a partially or completely managed-care model.

To some extent, Medicaid is the major program to help provide health care services to children of the poor. But in reality, Medicaid has never provided care to all children of limited means. Receipt of Medicaid had traditionally been linked to receipt of other governmental subsidies (such as Aid to Families of Dependent Children, AFDC), but earlier chapters have pointed out how welfare policy has changed recently, and this will in some ways affect access to Medicaid. Major changes in Medicaid were enacted in the late 1980s. Starting in 1987, Congress required states to extend Medicaid benefits to pregnant women and to children under age 6 with family incomes below 133% of the federal poverty income guidelines. From 1991 on, states were to cover all children under age 19 who were born after September 30, 1993, and whose family income was below 100% of the federal poverty level. Sometimes eligible children are not enrolled; in a recent study of Medicaid in various states estimated that about 30% of uninsured children nationally were eligible for Medicaid but not enrolled in 1995 (Cassil, 1997). The rest of the children, though uninsured, were not Medicaid eligible. Even the expansions in recent years and the new programs enacted to expand coverage to more children, such as the State Children's Health Insurance Program (SCHIP) (which can be administered through the traditional Medicaid program or through other special programs that states create, since states have great flexibility with the new legislation) will not necessarily cover all children (Hofferth, 1993). Beginning in 1997, more and more persons receiving welfare aid will be on limited years of eligibility and will be urged in many ways to enter the labor force. If these welfare changes decrease numbers of people receiving payments, the numbers of poor children on Medicaid may decline, but the numbers of near-poor children who may or may not receive health insurance coverage as part of the employment of a parent may increase.

Studies estimating the prevalence and length of gaps in health insurance coverage demonstrate that the Medicaid program even as structured before welfare reform, leaves many gaps, and the extent to which the new program will fill those gaps is unclear. Any switch to a state block grant system for Medicaid, as was discussed in the last few years, would probably leave even more gaps in coverage (Kogan et al., 1995; Maurer, 1993). In a follow-up 1991 survey of respondents to the 1988 National Maternal and Infant Health Survey (NMIHS), about one quarter of children were without health insurance for at least 1 month during their first 3 years of life. For half of these children, the gap was as long as 6 months. Overall, children from families with lower income, education, public insurance, earlier childbearing, and unstable marital status were those most likely to have a gap in insurance. The working poor (those families earning from $10,000 to $19,000 a year) experienced the highest level of gaps (Kogan et al., 1995). This group of families is likely to increase in numbers if welfare reform meets its goals of reducing the number of persons carried on public welfare rolls.

This study reinforces what we already know about the important links between poverty, limited income, and problems in attaining access to health care services. The number of children in poverty is estimated to have increased in the United States over the past 25 years (Chafel, 1993; Scarbrough, 1993). Over 14 million children in the United States are now poor. Their poverty is not evenly distributed across racial/ethnic groups but is disproportionately concentrated among members of minority groups. Overall, about one in every five American children live in families that are poor, but for African American children, 46% live in poverty, as do 40% of Latino children and 32% of Native American children, in contrast to only 12% of white children (Scarbrough, 1993).

Poor children experience an increased risk of poor health, poor nutrition, school failure and dropout, accidental injury and death, homelessness, and many other problems (Scarbrough, 1993). We need to remember that it is the children's families (and especially the adult or adults within them) whose circumstances lead to the poverty of the children. Parents in these families are generally less educated and have fewer job skills, and many have serious health problems, including substance abuse in some cases. Given the difficulty of solving the problem of poverty among these families (some of which experts argue is related to the need for more jobs and better paying jobs; Bergmann, 1994), provision of services to the children may be one of the better short-term solutions, one that avoids some of the political liabilities associated with other kinds of antipoverty programs (Bergmann, 1994). Though many policy analysts have focused on improved child care as one of the most important short-term solutions (Bergmann, 1994; Hofferth, 1993), others have focused on the need to protect the "human capital" of our society, including the health and vitality of children, as one of the most important aspects of human capital of any society (Watts, 1997).

The establishment of school-based clinics has recently been proposed as one small, but important, solution to improving poor children's living situations and opportunities to learn. One criticism of many programs that deal with health and social needs of children in the United States today is their fragmentation. A recent critique of such programs has argued that "the United States does not have a system of care for our children and families. Rather, we have a collection of activities and funding mechanisms that create a complex, fragmented patchwork of services and programs"(Grason & Guyer, 1995, p. 565). As was noted earlier in this book, the nation's initial response to the plight of children through the creation of the Children's Bureau was less fragmented but not long-lasting. Now over 300 separate programs are available that deal categorically with health, social, and educational needs of children (Grason & Guyer, 1995; National Commission on Children, 1991). Grason and Guyer (1995) have argued that children's health programs could benefit by having the structure of a single piece of legislation, analogous to the Older Americans Act (42 §3001) passed in 1965, which addressed in a consolidated fashion multiple aspects of services for the elderly (including some health care services, although not Medicare or Social Security). The overarching purpose of this act was to create a framework for a comprehensive system designed to assist older persons and thus to achieve integration of programs rather than separate piecemeal efforts. Although Title V of the Social Security Act (42 §301), the Maternal and Child Health Services Block Grant, might serve as the starting point for system reform, that is not occurring at this point in time and the current national trends are against consolidated efforts at the national level.

LITERATURE ON SCHOOL-BASED CLINICS

Patterns of Growth

A few school-based health clinics were started before the 1980s. The Cambridge Health Department began providing services in the elementary schools in the 1960s. The West Dallas Youth Center at Pinkston High School was begun in the late 1960s and was part of a federally funded experimental project in the 1970s (Kaplan, 1995; Passarelli, 1994). Beginning in the late 1970s and early 1980s, the Robert Wood Johnson Foundation began funded projects in four major cities: Chicago; Kansas City, Missouri; Flint, Michigan; and Houston. Since the 1980s, there has been some growth of school-based clinics, mostly in the form of primary health care centers in schools operated by local health agencies. These clinics began to pop up in different parts of the country, more or less serendipitously. The initial models tended to focus on adolescents and included a motive of prevention of teen pregnancy. Later, more comprehensive models were adopted whose goals were to help prevent substance abuse, depression, and sexually transmitted diseases and to provide access to primary health care services (Dryfoos, 1994). Many of these still focused on adolescents. In 1987, the Robert Wood Johnson Foundation funded more projects, almost all of which were located in high schools (Marks & Marzke, 1993). Now at least 12 states are helping to support the growth of various types of clinics within their states (Dryfoos, 1994).

The early efforts in school-based clinics began when national groups targeted access to medical services as the key barrier to better health for the adolescent population (Society for Adolescent Medicine, 1992). Studies concluded that those from 12 to 18 years of age faced barriers to health care access, lacked available services, and had low utilization rates (Lear et al., 1991). The rationale was that if adolescents would not go to health care services, then health care services must be brought to the youth. Because of the success of pilot projects, school-based health care clinics have grown (Dryfoos, 1994; Lear, 1991). Many of these clinics provide a wide range of services, including acute care treatment, birth control, counseling, anger management, and crisis intervention (Beilenson, Miola, & Farmer, 1995; Brindis, 1995; Santelli, Kouzis, & Newcomer, 1996).

Interest in school-based clinics has been slowly growing in a number of states. A review of school-based health centers in the early 1990s concluded that the numbers had grown from 31 in 1984 to 327 in 1991 to 415 school-based and 95 school-linked clinics in 1992 (Kaplan, 1995). The largest number of these served high schools (214). Another 53 were documented in middle and junior high schools and 79 in elementary schools. About 69 centers served a combination of kindergarten through high school students. Kaplan (1995) differentiated school-based health centers (school-based health clinics) from school-linked health centers (SLHCs) and differentiated both of them from traditional school health services. In contrast to traditional school services, both school-based health clinics and SLHCs provide on-site primary and preventive medical and mental health diagnostic and treatment services. school-based health clinics are those located in a school or on school grounds and usually serving only students in that school. SLHCs are health programs that have a formal written agreement with a school to provide health services to students at a site off school grounds. They may provide care to students attending a variety of schools as well as out-of-school youth. Generally, the school-linked services effort is part of a larger movement for more integration of education, health, and social services for children (Kaplan,

1995).

A more recent review of new models of health services delivery in the schools concluded that the greatest enrollment and number of users were still found in high schools and junior high schools and stated that in addition to a medically oriented staff member, there were often counseling personnel and, in over half the clinics, social workers also (Yates, 1994a). Earlier programs were heavily concentrated in high schools with a pregnancy prevention focus, but the models have now shifted to general medical care and psychosocial counseling, although those in high schools continue to have a focus on pregnancy prevention also. Growing numbers are located in middle schools and elementary schools, but these experiences are less well documented (Dryfoos, 1994). Among the most recently available data on numbers of programs are those from the Making the Grade project, a national grant program of the Robert Wood Johnson Foundation. The foundation reports 913 school-based clinics in 1996, up 50% from 2 years earlier ("Quick Updates", 1997). New York was the national leader with 149 centers, followed by Florida with 66. Most of these currently provide medical and mental health services to children within schools. The growth is attributed to some increased state funding, as well as support from community leaders, local schools, hospitals, and community health centers. During the 1995-96 school year, 34 states allocated almost $42 million in state and federal block grant funds to school-based centers ("Number," 1997).

Types of Services and Providers

More of the studies in the literature have dealt with adolescents and high school clinics (Balassone, Bell, & Peterfreund, 1991; Beilenson et al., 1995; Borenstein, Harvilchuck, Rosenthal, & Santelli, 1997; Brindis, Kapphahn, McCarter, & Wolfe, 1995; Fischer, Juszczark, Friedman, Schneider, & Chapar, 1992; Galavotti & Lovick, 1989; Harold & Harold, 1993; McCord, Klein, Foy, & Fothergill, 1993; 1995; Tokarski, 1995; Walter et al., 1996). Many of these have focused on specialized problems of reproductive health, human sexuality, alcohol and substance abuse counseling, and mental health issues as well as overall general health. These issues often generate the most controversy in communities and in the implementation stage. A 1995 review of school-based health clinics reported that the three major advocacy issues are provision of family planning and HIV services, delivery of mental health services, and funding (Klein & Cox, 1995). Some of these more controversial services are not needed in elementary schools, and the literature has not included as many examples of issues and concerns in the settings with younger children.

Some other examples of more specialized programs are those in rural areas and those dealing with mental health services. Rural adolescents appear unwilling to change their primary care site to a school-based health clinic but are willing to use services offered at the site on an episodic basis for acute medical care, miscellaneous services, and reproductive-related health services (Ricket, Davis,

& Ryan, 1997; Terwilliger, 1994). The availability of on-site mental health services in schools improves the access to these services and is particularly important in that schools are now mandated to provide services in regular school settings to many children with mental health problems (Flaherty, Weist, & Warner, 1996). In a pilot study that provided mental health services to high school students as part of a school-based clinic in Baltimore, treated students showed improvements in self-concept and decreased depression scores (Weist, Paskewitz, Warner, & Flaherty, 1996).

Several recent articles have discussed models of integrating access to health care services through school-based health clinics and traditional school health services. Terwilliger (1994) explored these issues with a special focus on rural schools and examined whether school-based health clinics are accessible as defined by four criteria of accessibility: available, community-based, affordable, and culturally acceptable. In the site that she examined in detail in a rural area of Pennsylvania, she found that school-based health clinics are accessible to children and families and have a high enrollment and usage rate.

Yates (1994b) has recently reviewed efforts in several different geographic locations in the United States. San Antonio has expanded its efforts into a more coordinated plan for its 60,000 students in 95 schools. They are now served by 66 registered nurses, six advanced nurse practitioners, 20 licensed vocational nurses and 28 health aides. Because of concerns about reproductive health care, the efforts were started with children in elementary school in the 1989-90 school year. The clinic was named a pediatric extension clinic and focused on children with minor illnesses who were attending school, children with long-term disabilities who did not keep doctor's appointments, and children with untreated psychoeducational, behavioral disorders. Over the next few years, additional clinics were added in three more schools, and by the 1992-93 school year, the duties of the six advanced nurse practitioners were rearranged to allow for primary care activities such as Early, Periodic, Screening, Diagnosis and Treatment (EPSDT) screens and clinics at five additional elementary schools. There are also school-linked clinics funded at community agencies in several locations.

In Baltimore County, Maryland, wellness centers were started initially in one high school in a high-need area and then expanded to a center that cared for children of high school students and also to a middle school. In January 1994, one was opened in an elementary school and funded from Medicaid billings. One limitation found in several of the Baltimore clinics was that students were more knowledgeable about the availability of sports physicals and reproductive health services at the centers than they were about other services. Students in two middle and high school clinics identified the two major barriers to use of the services as difficulty in obtaining permission from a classroom teacher to leave class to attend the clinic and the requirement of parental permission for students to use services (Keyl, Hurtado, Barber, & Burton, 1996).

Several recent articles have focused on who is best able to staff school-based health centers. Overall, most are staffed by nurse practitioners, some of whom have received training as family nurse practitioners and others of whom are pediatric nurse practitioners (Rajsky-Steed, 1996; Urbinati, Steele, Harter, & Harrell, 1996). A few training programs have created a specialization of school nurse practitioners so that there are available nurses with specialized training to deal with both the health issues of younger children in elementary schools and the adolescent health issues of high school aged students (Urbinati et al., 1996).

Funding Issues and State Examples

In the early 1990s, the chairman of the House Committee on Government Operations requested the General Accounting Office (GAO) to look into the issue of how school-based health centers could expand access to health care services for both adolescents and younger children who had limited access to care and to explore the financial and other obstacles that school-based health clinics must overcome. The GAO completed case studies at eight school-based health clinics in three states: New York, California, and New Mexico (*School-Based Health Centers*, 1994). Four of the case studies were conducted in high schools, two in a middle school and a high school/middle school combination, and two in elementary schools (one in San Jose, California, and the other in New York City). The GAO found a lack of stable financing to be a major problem with the centers. State, local, and private funds supplied most of the funding. If federal funds were used, the funds were generally reimbursement from the Medicaid program or grants from the Maternal and Child Health Block Grant. In general, only a small amount of funding (2%) came from payments by students enrolled in school-based health clinics or private insurers. Other common concerns were problems recruiting and retaining appropriately trained nurse practitioners and physician assistants and debates about the appropriateness of providing reproductive health services in the high schools.

A different article that examined two schools in Baton Rouge, Louisiana and one in New Orleans that were part of the Robert Wood Johnson projects reported that sustained funding for these was still a question, although the state was providing some planning grant monies for new ones through federal dollars (Yates, 1994). Clinics related to specific situations of local and state laws in Seattle and Dallas were also described. The author concluded that "the vision of an integrated seamless system of health care services in the school ... seems still a dream" (p. 36). Over and over again, it is apparent from the literature that continued funding is often a serious issue and that approaches and solutions vary from place to place. A school health telephone survey conducted in 40 major metropolitan areas reported that only 42% of clinics contacted were successfully billing for some services (Hacker, Fried, Bablouzian, & Roeber, 1994).

Dryfoos(1994), in a book about a transition from school-based clinics to full-service schools, described two schools that come close to that vision as well as reviewing 10 early school-based clinics. She concluded that no single school-based clinic model had emerged during this developmental stage. Public heath departments and community health clinics were the most frequent sponsors, followed by hospitals or medical schools, community-based organizations and school districts themselves. Less comprehensive programs were more likely to be run by the schools themselves than by health-related agencies. Her two models of full-service schools were a middle school in Washington Heights, New York, that in essence ran a settlement house within the auspices of the school and a middle school in Modesto, California, in which a new school campus was built to house a middle school and a county library branch, located adjacent to a Salvation Army recreation center that was a neighborhood-based agency for youth. The school included a case management approach to social services that took health services funded through a state Healthy Starts Initiative.

Dryfoos (1994) included an appendix that described 12 different state efforts up to 1994. The states discussed were: Arkansas, California, Connecticut, Florida, Georgia, Kentucky, Massachusetts, Michigan, New Jersey, New Mexico, New York, and Oregon. One important issue in each state was the extent to which state funds were provided to create a more secure financial base for projects. In some, innovative programs were tried but not expanded over time. In others, the issue of legislation had been resolved but not funding for programs, and changes in state leadership and budgets made the future of some programs questionable.

Three large initiatives (relative to the size of the states) were in Arkansas, California, and New York. In Arkansas in 1987, the then-director of the Arkansas Department of Health, Joycelyn Elders, encouraged communities to apply for grants for primary health care services in schools. Over the next 2 years, 26 enhanced school health services clinics were set up in elementary, middle and high schools in the state. The school clinic staff were employees of the state health department, although the legislation passed by the Arkansas legislature in 1991 ensured that no school-based clinic could be placed in a public school without a request signed by the local school board of directors. Funding was from a grant from the Arkansas Indigent Health Advisory Council, the Annie Casey Foundation, Medicaid reimbursement funds, the Child Health Block Grant, and $786,000 funded through the Arkansas Department of Health as of 1993.

California had had many clinics funded through private grants. Then a major state initiative was begun under Governor Wilson in 1991, but the funding was cut back from $20 million in 1992 to $13 million in 1993. Elaborate plans to include a new nonprofit agency, the Foundation Consortium on School-Linked Services to help in monitoring and technical assistance was also planned, but these efforts were all vulnerable to variations in state funding. In New York, what became the first statewide school-based clinic initiative was started as the School Health Demonstration Project in 1981 in response to legislation developed by the Black and Puerto Rican Caucus. There are now over 140 school-based clinics. Much of this is now being supported by special state and federal project grants and the Maternal and Child Health Block Grant. The use of these block grant funds has created a more stable funding environment for many of these programs.

In some states, much of the effort to establish school-based clinics has been linked with adolescent health initiatives. In Connecticut, school-based clinics grew out of teen pregnancy prevention initiatives. In 1987, the Department of Health Services offered small planning grants to four communities and then funded clinics in several places. That same year, a line item of half a million dollars was appropriated for school-based health services in the state budget. The state made these clinics a high priority, and by mid-1993 it had funded 19 and had 8 more in planning stages. Clinics are also expected to be certified as Medicaid providers. Michigan has been funding 19 centers since 1990. All centers must have 20% local funds for matching. Most of their programs are connected with other teen programs, and the issue of funding remains, because some local funds must be raised each year. In New Mexico, as in Michigan, most of the centers are part of adolescent health efforts of the state health department, and funding is from Medicaid as well as from the Maternal and Child Health Block Grant.

The Florida effort was part of the legislative push of Governor Lawton Chiles to move to full-service schools. This legislation required the state board of education and department of health and rehabilitative services to jointly establish programs to serve high risk students in need of medical and social services. The full-service dollars go to county school districts, which then subcontract with other agencies. This effort is funded partially by state appropriations and partially by a special tax on athletic, exercise, and physical fitness facilities and clubs. The Georgia effort began more modestly, with a one-time surplus of funds in 1987 that was used to fund some model programs. Special legislation and a named program have not been part of the effort in Georgia. Most of the funds for the programs currently come from Medicaid, the Maternal and Child Health Block Grant, other categorical state funds for pregnancy prevention or substance abuse prevention and some private foundations. In Kentucky, especially from a clinical services side, the effort was much slower. The initial programs in Kentucky were really focused on helping local agencies to coordinate their services through the use of school sites and to make them more accessible. Funding was provided by the department of education in the state and the cabinet for human resources. This part of the effort was large, with a budget of almost $16 million in 1993 and 223 centers serving 414 schools. Twenty sites are now funding health programs as well, with funding from the maternal and child health division of the health department, but the health aspect is not the major part of the Kentucky initiative.

In Massachusetts, some early efforts were started in the mid-1980s. There is now a program linking centers in Massachusetts with a community facility and movement toward a development of community health networks in 27 regions. The Boston Board of Education and Department of Health os working out its own collaborative arrangements in the city. Before the introduction of managed care into the Massachusetts Medicaid program, some clinics were receiving almost a quarter of their operating expenses from Medicaid funds (Hacker, 1996). In 1992, Massachusetts received permission to funnel Medicaid recipients into managed care. The Medicaid funds for school-based clinics began to decline. With the assistance of the departments of medical assistance and public health, a number of clinics have been able to arrange for reimbursement for some services, generally for urgent or minor care.

Oregon started some clinics as early as 1984 and the state was supporting six by 1988, with counties picking up more. A cutback in the state budget in 1993 led to fears that all funding would be cut off. Although state funding of 11 clinics did remain, the funding picture as in some other states, remains questionable and variable from year to year.

One common strategy of many of these states that are looking for ways to achieve some fiscal stability is to tap into Medicaid funds and have the clinics become Medicaid providers and be reimbursed on a fee-for-service model for care or at least for certain special services such as EPSDT required screening. In 1991, Medicaid was providing only 2% of the operating costs of school-based clinics (Schlitt, Rickett, Montgomery, & Lear, 1995). The 24 school-based health centers that received support from the Robert Wood Johnson Foundation in 1992-93 reported that 13% of their operating budgets were received from patient care revenue, mostly Medicaid (Schlitt et al., 1995). An obstacle in many states to receipt of Medicaid funds is the lack of familiarity of the state Medicaid officials with school-based clinics. The most common reimbursement is for EPSDT examinations. In some states, such as Connecticut and Delaware, arrangements for Medicaid funds have been very difficult. After 3 years of discussion with the state Medicaid agency, the Connecticut Public Health Department continued to have difficulty acquiring reimbursement for primary care. In Delaware, the Medicaid program would not reimburse for school-based health centers during 1996. In contrast, in New Jersey and North Carolina, reimbursements are provided if clinics are sponsored by health care organizations already receiving Medicaid funding (Lear, Montgomery, Schlitt, & Rickett, 1996).

A serious potential problem for stable funding for Arizona school-based clinics is that Arizona is the first state to have an all-managed-care Medicaid program. Recent reports from more established school-based health centers in other states have reported drops in reimbursement dollars as managed care Medicaid grows in a state. For example, in 1994, the Baltimore City Health Department witnessed declines in Medicaid revenues of 35% for its school-based health centers as a result of managed care ("School Based Health Centers," 1994). Ones in the Bronx in the same year suffered a loss of $30,000. Minnesota, the state that has the largest percentage of the population enrolled in managed care and that has put major efforts into developing school-based clinics, has focused on trying to develop linkages between managed care and school-based programs. Healthy Start is a nonprofit health care organization in Minnesota that now covers all of the St. Paul high schools, with Title V Maternal and Child Health Block Grant funds as its major funding base, but that source of funds is capped. Healthy Start is exploring how to work with plans—in a shared or satellite primary care model—or as an independent primary care gatekeeper (Zimmerman & Reif, 1995). School-based health clinics have great difficulty negotiating with managed-care plans as individual sites of care unless the state is participating in development of relationships between managed-care plans and school-based clinics (Schlitt et al., 1995). As states beginning in 1998 are no longer required to obtain waivers to implement managed-care Medicaid programs, managed care will become more and more common in state Medicaid programs, creating more financial barriers for school-based health clinics.

Schools and health care providers running clinics in schools need to learn from the experiences of others. One sign of a growing trend is the recent creation of the National Assembly on School-Based Health Clinics. This group now sponsors an annual meeting (the first was held in Washington, DC in the summer of 1995) and has a newsletter, *Joining Hands* (McLean, Virginia), that can provide information to clinics starting out, as well as to those that have been underway for some period of time. Learning from the experience of other clinics is important for all new efforts, and experiences from clinics in Arizona may help in future development of school-based clinics.

CHAPTER 5

EXPERIENCES IN ARIZONA

The Development of New Clinics in a State with a Managed-Care Medicaid System

This chapter will first apply some specific models of school-based clinics to eight of the nine Flinn-funded projects within Arizona (the project that did not include school-based services is not discussed in this chapter). Then it will review in some detail those selected Arizona projects and the evaluations of their initial efforts. Finally, it will report the numbers of clinics and summarize the current situation in the state of Arizona with school-based clinics and will discuss some lessons from the experience in this one state.

MODELS OF SCHOOL-BASED CLINICS IN ARIZONA AND THEIR EVALUATION

This portion of the chapter will present some different models of school-based clinics, based both on the experiences of some specific Arizona projects and the experiences of other places as reported in the literature. It will also explain how a subset of the new projects in Arizona was evaluated and will categorize these evaluations.

One issue that became clearer as some of the projects developed was that most of these projects were more than school-based clinics. In fact, the foundation that was funding the projects required a health partner as well as a school or school district to be involved. As some of the projects developed, many formed community coalitions or boards also. One recent article on coalitions defined a coalition as an organization of individuals representing diverse organizations, factions, or constituencies that agree to work together to achieve a common goal

(Butterfoss, Goodman, & Wandersman, 1993). The coalition approach is part of a theoretical approach in health known as the social ecology approach. This approach argues that the individual is embedded in and influenced or supported by numerous groups and/or systems and that emphasizing only the individual and family risk factors about risk for unhealthy behaviors is too limited.

In her book advocating for full-service schools, Dryfoos (1994) talked about three different categories of projects, although she concluded that each of the 12 state efforts described in Appendix A of her book was unique in many ways. The first approach was a health clinic based in schools that delivered primary health care, psychosocial counseling and health education and was operated by a health department, hospital, or community health center. The second included youth services or family service centers, generally based in schools, that offered health, mental health, and family counseling, drug and alcohol counseling, recreation, and employment services, parenting education and/or child care on site and/or through linkages with other community agencies. The third type was a youth or family center that provided coordination with and referral to community agencies. Dryfoos's concept of the full-service school was adopted from efforts in Florida that defined a specific definition for a full service school. "A full-service school integrates education, medical, social and or human services that are beneficial to meeting the needs of children and youth and their families on school grounds or in locations which are easily accessible. A full-service school provides the types of prevention, treatment and support services children and families need to succeed." (Dryfoos, 1994, p. 142). Dryfoos stressed that services must be of high quality and comprehensive. The legislation recommends interagency partnerships that link the state with local public and private entities. As Dryfoos (1994) pointed out about most of the schools whose programs she reviewed, few programs operate at such a high level of integration. This is certainly true overall of the programs in Arizona.

I propose a modification of Dryfoos's typology to apply to the Flinn projects in Arizona (see Table 5.1). My own three categories are expansive projects, case management projects, and limited projects.

The limited model in the Dryfoos approach included primary care, psychosocial services, and health education services but not the complete range of expanded services. My definition of limited as used in the Flinn projects is more limited than Dryfoos's in that it refers to projects that had a focus mostly on primary care, with limited referrals to other types of services, such as dental care or very modest health education efforts. Two of the three projects that I would categorize as limited were limited as well in terms of the amount of time that the provider spent in the school; in one case the provider worked a full week, but not in just one or two schools, rather dividing his or her time across a number of schools.(Phoenix 1)

Expansive includes large-scale projects that were initially intended to provide a broader range of social and health services than the primary care, short-term acute health care that could be provided by a physician or nurse practitioner. The names of the provider institutions and the specific school districts are not identified in this book, although the report to the Flinn Foundation identifies specific school districts and partner provider institutions, as do reports from the Arizona Department of Health Services (Arizona Department of Health Services, 1997; Kronenfeld, 1996). The Southern Arizona 1, 3 and 4 projects with their evolving model of integration with Family Resource and Wellness Centers (FRWCs) clearly fit into this approach. As it has developed, the Phoenix 3 project may or may not fit into this category, but at least initially there was a broader goal and approach.

TABLE 5.1 Application of Dryfoos's Categories to Selected Arizona Projects

Categories	Flinn Projects
Expansive	Southern Arizona 1, 3 and 4
	Phoenix 3 (in initial intent)
Case-Management	Phoenix 4
Limited	Phoenix 2
	Phoenix 1
	Southern Arizona 2

*less perfect fit expansive model in initial design.

As described by Dryfoos, the case management model involves coordination with community-based services. In health services research more generally, *case management* usually refers to the coordination of the care of an individual and the management of care patterns and sources of care for that person. Given the presence of a managed-care Medicaid model in the state, the Arizona Health Care Cost Containment System (AHCCCS), the goal of the case management approach in the Flinn study (explained in more detail under Phoenix 4) was to enable the school nurse to have her more routine health care duties assumed by a nurse's aide so that the nurse could devote more of her time to managing the care of students and especially to helping those already on AHCCCS or possibly AHCCCS eligible to use their provider or get onto the system. For those for whom AHCCCS was not an option, a nurse practitioner from the hospital partner would be available at the school a limited number of hours, and the charity clinic at the hospital partner would also be a care option.

Most of the Flinn projects would be characterized as school based rather than school linked. The distinction is not always clear, however. This is true in these projects also. In some of the southern Arizona projects, the site for care is connected with the school district but is not necessarily a part of a currently functioning school within one of the area school districts.

I have also categorized these projects according to whether the health care provider or the school district seems to have played a larger role in initiation and then success of the project (Table 5.2). Examining this dimension in more detail may provide clues for the success of future projects. But because the projects are not static, this dimension is more subject to change as projects develop and change than the dimensions of categorization in Table 5.1. Table 5.2 shows my initial categorization of the relative role of the partners. I view the health care provider as playing the most important role in the initiation of projects Phoenix 1 and 2.

TABLE 5.2 Categorization of Projects by The Strength of the Initial Role of Each Health Partner as Compared to the School Partner in Beginning the Project

Categories	Projects
More Important Role For Health Partner	Phoenix 1
	Phoenix 2
Equal Role for Each	Southern Arizona 1
	Southern Arizona 2
More Important Roles for School District	Southern Arizona 3
	Southern Arizona 4
	Phoenix 3
	Phoenix 4

More equal roles between the two partners were the case for Southern Arizona 2 and the earlier phases of Southern Arizona 1. The other two Southern Arizona projects (3 and 4) and Phoenix 3 and 4 were, in my judgment, led more by the school at the initiation stage.

There could be some other ways to categorize projects, such as the consistency of the provider (in being the same person each time or a varying person), whether the clinic views itself as a free service or one in which a fee should be charged, whether the clinic is open to anyone in the school or only to those without health insurance, and whether the provider spends almost all of his or her time providing these types of services to schools, or does this as a small part of a broader health care delivery role. These types of factors are reviewed in the specific discussion of each project but are not employed to create a typology of projects.

Many different models of evaluations have been presented in the literature. One of the best known in the health care area is Donabedian's (1980) model of process, structure and outcome in which process evaluations addresses what has actually happened and what specific things have been done; structure evaluation addresses whether the approach itself is appropriate and is likely in the long run to produce the appropriate goals; and outcome evaluation addresses the actual (generally longer-term) outcomes or end results of a program or project. Evaluations can also be categorized as needs assessments, process evaluations, and impact assessments (Kirby, 1992). Kirby viewed needs assessments as those that assist in program development by identifying and demonstrating needs; process evaluation as a monitoring and assessment of the program services, with a focus in school-based clinics on clinic utilization, compliance with care and user satisfaction; and final stage, impact assessment, as similar to outcome evaluation, focusing on evaluating the impact and effectiveness of the program through such variables as improvements in health behaviors, decreases in risk taking, and improvements in attendance at the school. Kirby viewed these different types of evaluations as most appropriate at different stages of the development of a school clinic. Typically, needs assessments answer questions either before a clinic opens or during the first year of the operation. Process evaluations have to be carried out after clinics are open but are best if designed during the planning stages of the project. Impact assessments cannot be conducted until after clinics are open but are best conducted after programs have been implemented and any initial modifications have occurred in the program. Often, this takes 3 or more years of clinic operations.

In the Arizona projects, as in many real-life projects that involve the community and other institutions (in this case, schools), neat models of evaluation became less clear and less simple as the actual operational processes began. Although I participated in the design of an evaluation of a number of new clinics started with funding from the Flinn Foundation, as often happens with the creation of new projects, things did not begin on the schedules initially planned. Rather than being able to keep to a proposed time schedule, most of the projects could not begin their clinics as initially planned. Many visits occurred for the collection of qualitative and observational data, but actual operations of clinics varied across several years. Moreover, as interest in school-based clinics in Arizona grew, the foundation began a new second group of projects a year after the initial ones. Even in the projects started in the first year of the grant, only two were able to have much of their plan for getting the clinic into operation implemented during the first year of the project. In fact, different projects have quite different histories. Most of this evaluation examines issues of process and structure, not outcomes.

FOUNDATION-FUNDED ARIZONA PROJECTS

Phoenix 1

This project has a different history and background than many of the other projects, for most of the other projects began in response to the Flinn Fund solicitation for child or adolescent health projects. This one was not part of the group of projects funded in the first year but was added after a false start with a different project that included the hospital. The initial goal of this project was a clinic for elementary school children in five schools in a larger school district in the Phoenix metropolitan area. A nurse practitioner connected with the hospital had previously begun a clinic with one elementary school in the district. The project expanded into five schools aided by a 12-month grant to cover the period from June 1, 1994, through May 30, 1995.

One unusual aspect of this project was the strong preexisting ties between the hospital that was the provider organization and its affiliated private foundation and the surrounding community. The hospital was founded with a mission of service to that community and runs a number of projects, mostly through its foundation, that demonstrate that commitment to the community. Thus, this was not a partnership newly created to obtain external grant support. For example, the hospital had been funding snacks at several of the schools for years. Before the grant, the hospital was providing services at a school-based clinic at one school with which they had developed a partnership. Also, a pediatrician with the hospital had provided some free care before the nurse practitioner began to provide services.

The school district that is part of this project is much larger than the community that the hospital has historically helped and contains 26 elementary schools and three junior high schools. The schools range from quite poor to more affluent, although most of the five served by this project are among the poorer schools in the district. The composition of the population in the school district is changing, with growing numbers of Asian and Hispanic students. The proportion of children on free or reduced lunches ranges from 20% to 93%. The number of children who do not speak English in their homes is also growing. In one school, seven different languages are spoken in the homes of the children, and the school maintains a large English as a Second Language (ESL) program, with 34% of the students in the school enrolled in it. In another school, Spanish is the major second language, and one third of the children are in an ESL program for that language.

This project fits a more limited model in terms of the total range of services, since the hospital is providing a nurse practitioner to go into the schools for a half day to a day a week. No goal for this to evolve into a family and community resources center model exists, but the school district itself does provide social workers, and many of the schools run extra feeding programs, summer recreational programs in collaboration with the city recreation department, and special after-school programs. The hospital does maintain a program that provides some nutrition supplement as part of the efforts of its foundation.

One unusual strength of this project has been the nurse practitioner's interest in data collection. A computerized data collection system has been used for each encounter, providing excellent-quality data (Wenzel, 1996), some of which is summarized here. Of the respective projects, Phoenix 1 reported the highest number of encounters with the nurse practitioner, with over 2,000 encounters in a 1-year period. The patients seen at the project tended to be young, with over 75%

in Grade 4 or below. A full third, or 34%, of the patients were in either preschool or kindergarten.

Gender was split in a 51% male to 49% female ratio. Ethnicity was divided among three categories, with Anglos (non-Hispanic whites) and Hispanics making up 48.1% and 43.4% of encounters, respectively. The remaining 8.5%, composing an "other" category, included African Americans, Native Americans, Asians, and others. The most commonly reported language spoken in the home for this project was English, at 57.4%. The Spanish language was reported in 34.9% of the encounters, and the "other" category (mostly Asian languages) made up the remaining 7.7%.

This project reported a free- or reduced-lunch status variable for 94% of the encounters. Given that one of the schools has a low percentage of its student body on free or reduced lunch (about 20%), the overwhelming use of the clinic by students with greater economic needs indicates that the clinic is reaching the students who most need its services, rather than the smaller proportion of middle-class students that may be present in some of the schools. This has been possible even though (at the insistence of the nurse practitioner and in contrast to some other projects) the clinic will treat any student who wishes to receive care, without attempting to determine whether he or she has private health care insurance or is on an AHCCCS plan.

Some children used the clinic over and over again, although most did not. The highest number of encounters reported for a single individual was 14. Seven individuals were seen 10 or more times, and 13 were seen from 5 to 9 times. Thus, while a few students are very high utilizers of the clinic, most usage is distributed among a wide number of students.

The most commonly reported health problem was earache and related problems (31.8% of all problems). The other category, which included immunizations and well-child visits, was the next most commonly reported value, at 30.1 percent. The remaining major problem categories were cold (including cough), sore throat, skin, asthma, tooth, and injury. In 13.2% of the encounters, a second problem was reported.

Only 188 (8.9% of the encounters resulted in a referral. Dental was the largest referral category, with 85 referrals, or 45.2% of all referrals. A dental referral was made in 4% of all visits. Physician referrals were made in 73 encounters, or 3.5% of all visits, and the remaining referrals (16%) were divided among social workers, therapists, and other providers. The number of referrals to nonproject physicians was greater among Anglos than among Hispanics or the composite "other" category, perhaps indicating a difference in insurance coverage. Dental referrals were far more common among Hispanics than among the Anglos, indicating greater problems of unmet need for dental care in that group. Only children with greater need for dental care were referred according to the nurse practitioner because the dental care providers that were part of the Hospital Foundation did not want to see only children from this project.

Compared to many of the other projects, this has been a smooth-running and successful program. Several factors, both personal and structural, are important in the success of its operation. First, an important personal factor is that the individual nurse practitioner is very committed and dedicated to the success of the project. That enthusiasm carries over to the principals and school nurses and increases the buy-in to the project at all levels within the schools. Moreover, this enthusiasm seems to have been conveyed to the overall administration of the hospital, for commitment to the project is strong at the highest levels of operation of the hospital.

An important structural factor is the preexisting commitment of the hospital to the community and the prior relationship with one of the elementary schools. Thus, the hospital had a positive image in the community from the beginning, and one of the school principals already knew and had worked with the hospital and its administration. This helped to smooth the incorporation of this project into the school district and also seemed to be an important factor that other principals mentioned for wanting to be part of the project. Many of them had previously talked with the principal of the local elementary school and were enthusiastic about being involved in a collaborative project with the hospital. The personal and structural interact, of course. Because the nurse practitioner on the project was well liked by students, the principals, and the school nurses, the strong positive image of the hospital was reinforced within the new schools by his success, leading to generally smooth incorporation of the projects into the schools in most cases.

One major strength of this project is the strong relationship with the hospital and its foundation and the backup that provides for extra services, such as referrals if needed. In addition, some medications are supplied by the hospital and handed out by the nurse practitioner free of charge. Laboratory work and even x-ray work and surgical care for two children with special needs during the first year of the project were also provided. The strong ties with the hospital's group of pediatricians and other specialists provided a backup network of services for the children and made the clinic (although limited in the amount of time spent in any one school and in the overall model) more able than some of the other projects to provide a full range of physical health services to the children.

All projects can improve, and one of the issues that the nurse practitioner targeted for improvement was to gain better knowledge of how many children the different physicians at the hospital might be willing to see. This would help the nurse practitioner plan referrals for some more serious health problems. Another was to improve the availability on site of certain clinical services, such as hemoglobins and cultures. The hospital bought a machine to perform hemoglobins on site and started providing culture kits for strep tests on site. Another issue was dental care. The foundation does maintain a children's dental clinic where the children can be seen for $15 a visit. During the first year of this project, the dental clinic saw 1,271 children, and 90 of these had been referred by the nurse practitioner. The need for dental care could quickly overwhelm the clinic, and the nurse practitioner feels constrained to refer only the most serious dental cases, even though many more children have dental health problems.

One weakness in the project is at the top administrative level within the district. This is a large elementary school district, and the support both from the superintendent and from the board has not been consistent. It is not so much that the board has opposed the project as that the board has had a number of problems. Due to these, it is difficult to ascertain support for a relatively small project in only one part of a much larger district. There were board elections in the fall of the first year of operation of the grant. A new superintendent had strong support from the staff but not with the new board. In fact, that superintendent left the district as the initial phases of the project ended, creating even less clarity about administrative support at the top of the district. In the first year of operation, there was great concern about cutbacks in the district budgets and even, at one point, a concern that school nurses might be eliminated or seriously cut back at many of the elementary schools. By the end of the school year, this had not happened but it did lower morale. On the more positive side, the lease agreement with the school districts was renegotiated for 5 years, and that length of the contract has been taken by the hospital and the people from the hospital and the school involved with the school-based clinic as a show of commitment for the project.

This issue of the administrative structure within the district reinforces that this project is dominated by the hospital. It is the hospital's commitment that allows the project to continue. Although grant support from the Flinn Foundation has ended, the nurse practitioner is continuing to provide care on a very similar schedule to the one before, with funding from the hospital and its foundation. One strength of this project is the willingness of the hospital and foundation together to commit a full-time person to the school-based clinics. In the summer, the nurse practitioner does other work for the hospital, but otherwise he devotes almost all time to the project. Thus, he has had time to create and manage a database and to conduct home visits occasionally. The presence of one person with a full-time commitment to the project is a strength in the eyes of school personnel and allows the nurse practitioner to have a strong sense of accomplishment and ownership of the project that does not occur if personnel are spending some time on a school-based clinic and some on regular clinical or other responsibilities.

This project has a strong likelihood of continuing because of the commitment of the hospital. Both its commitment and the fortunate choice of a provider who has turned out to have many skills (a strong clinician, liked by nurses, administrators, and children, with a strong interest in maintaining a database, a good relationship with hospital personnel for referrals and support, and the ability to work hard and see a large number of children over the year) are important. This project demonstrates that for success, at least one of the two parties needs strong support at high administrative levels. The turmoil within the district administration during the first year of operation could have led to the failure of the project, but the commitment of the hospital to the community and the positive attitude of the nurse practitioner at the schools kept this problem from becoming a major obstacle. The enthusiasm of the nurse practitioner helped to maintain enthusiasm at the individual school level, even when the positions of the school nurses were threatened by budget concerns in the district. The district political and administrative leadership appears to be growing more stable, thus enhancing the chances that this successful project will continue.

Phoenix 2

This project was initially funded as a 13-month joint effort of a Phoenix-based hospital, especially its family medicine center, and a nearby school district. The two groups had already worked together, and a resident had spent some time in one specific school as part of a community medicine rotation before applying for the Flinn funding. The project placed a resident physician in the school each Monday to work with the school health nurse and function as a physician for acute needs, health histories, and physical exams. The project also had initial goals of gathering information on medical problems facing the underserved in this area and providing education to school nurses. This project was one of the few to actually start operations close to its initially planned time, primarily because the residents had already worked in the school in the previous year.

The school was a K-through-3 elementary school that was undergoing rapid growth, from 520 students 6 years earlier to 950 the first year of the project. The racial composition of the school changed from predominantly white to majority minority. The neighborhood included many rental apartments and subsidized Section 8 housing, resulting in a 43% turnover rate in school enrollment. Most children were poor, with 90% on free or reduced lunch. About 40% of the school was Anglo, with the rest a mix of ethnicities, in which Hispanics predominated. This was not a resource-rich school. For example, no social workers were employed by the school district, although the nurse and principal had, on occasion, conducted home visits in the past.

The principal of the school has been working to bring other resources into the school with some success, as her vision is for the school to be a center for community resources for the parents and children. Besides the school-based clinic, two counselors, a social worker intern from a local university, a school psychologist, and volunteer coordinator are now available. Thus, although, I view this project as a limited project both in overall concept and in the amount of time the clinic is in operation, that is a more apt description of the role of the hospital than the total vision of the principal. The clinic is open only one morning a week. The residents focus on physical health problems, although the principal in the school has been interested in this project because of her awareness of the relation between health and the ability to concentrate on academics.

I have also characterized this as a project in which the provider has played a more major role than the school. This was a difficult assessment to make for it was the principal who initially contacted the hospital to figure out how to acquire help for the children in the school. As this inquiry was conveyed to the family practice residency director, however, the role of the hospital became more important both in sending residents to the school and in applying for Flinn funds. The residency has incorporated the school experience as an important part of exposure to medical care outside of a hospital and office context.

This project was the only one to incorporate the design of the school-based clinic into an ongoing residency program. Almost all care is provided by second- and third-year family practice residents as part of their community medicine rotation. Often the same resident will come for a month, providing some continuity. Although there are advantages and disadvantages to the incorporation of a services delivery project into a residency training program, one advantage is that the health care provider is also receiving a direct benefit from participation in the program. The students are receiving an educational experience in a different community setting, something required by many residency programs. Thus, it will be in the best interests of both the school district and the hospital to continue the program.

Overall, the operation of the clinic has moved along smoothly. Parental permissions have been obtained, and numbers have grown as new students have enrolled in the school. Residents respond quite positively about their experience at the school and are excited by the amount of direct patient contact they receive. Generally, the clinic has been busy. The school nurse is an important link in triaging patients and having enough students available each week but not so many as to be overwhelming to the residents. This has generally worked well. Both teachers and parents are now supportive of the project and indicate that they do not want it to end.

Three different sets of data were collected: data from visits to residents in both 1994-95 and 1993-94 and data from all of the encounters with the school nurse in 1993-94. During the 1994-95 school year, this project reported 359 visits, an increase from the 220 visits of the first year of operation. Considering that the clinic was only open 1 day a week, the total number of students seen was substantial. Using the Year 2 data, the majority of the students were Anglos (44.6%), followed by Hispanics (36.2%), African Americans (11.1%), and "others" (8.1%). Most patients received either a free (79.4%) or a reduced (3.6%) lunch. The most commonly seen health problems were earache (15%), skin problem (13.4%) or sore throat (13.1%). Other common problems were coughs (10.9%), colds (7.5%), and general aches (7%). In both years, medications were provided in almost 40% of the encounters.

During the 1993-94 school year, total reported nurse-only visits numbered 5,979. Boys were seen in 61.2% of all encounters, probably due to the high number of visits by boys for medications. As other school health literature has reported, boys are more likely to use drugs such as Ritalin to control attention deficit hyperactivity disorder (ADHD). ADHD management was a major activity for the school nurse. Besides visits for medications, accidental injuries were the most common problem presented, followed by stomachaches, skin problems, headaches, and lice.

In addition to the school-based clinic plans of the grant, the project in its initial proposal planned to gather information on the medical problems facing the underserved in this area and to provide education to the school nurses. These were harder goals to achieve. Though some education of the school nurses did occur, no data on its impact were collected. Nor was information on problems facing the underserved obtained in any systematic manner, although residents did conduct some health education classes for the elementary school children.

There have been few problems. Give the acute, short-term nature of most of the problems brought into the clinic, the rotation of residents has not been a problem, although lack of continuity of care is one potential limitation of this model. Though some residents were initially apprehensive about the types of students and their abilities, most now feel comfortable with the school setting. At times, it is necessary to have someone available to interpret for younger students who do not speak English and for some parents, for most residents have not been bilingual. Both secretaries at the school are bilingual and have interpreted as needed.

The most important limitation is the lack of referral sources for seriously ill children, as the hospital does not maintain a large indigent care fund and the residency is part of a family practice residency, not a pediatrics residency. Serious problems of the children require hospitalization at a larger hospital or the specialized children's hospital in the city. The hospital and practice have been able to see a few children who have needed referrals. For a few serious cases, children and their parents have been referred to one of two larger hospitals that have such a fund. Occasionally, the clinic has used all its sample medications and has been left with none available to give to the parents of the child, a source of frustration to both the residents and parents of the children.

Now that the project has entered a new phase without Flinn Foundation funding, some new ideas have occurred to both the hospital and the school district. There is now an active community association that is working with the school, and they are interested in whether there might be a way to have a clinic open to more than just the school-age children, perhaps to serve older and younger siblings and parents of the children as well as other adults in the neighborhood.

Although there has been a brief discussion about whether the residents might come more than once a week, overall the school believes that once a week has worked out well. They have conducted some follow-up with children. If there is a problem that develops as part of treatment, parents mat bring the child to the clinic with the doctor's practice affiliated with the residency, which is only a few blocks away. This helps to eliminate the need for more time in the school. The hospital has provided some in-service education programs to school nurses in other schools as well this year.

The project has agreed to some expansions. A pharmacy will be provided that should help solve the issue of lack of sample medications, and the hospital has made a commitment as part of community outreach to support the efforts in the overall school district and to keep certain stocks of prescription drugs available free for some children that cannot afford them. Discussion of expanding to other schools within the district has begun. An ongoing discussion between the hospital and the school is the role of the outside provider who is at the clinic once a week. Is it reasonable to expect that person to become a continuous provider? Should the person be an adjunct to the school and help to set up referral networks? If extra help is needed, how can it be obtained beyond the residents?

From the perspective of resident education, the expectations of the hospital have been met and exceeded. The residents know much more about schoolchildren and the problems of managing children in school. They have learned to think about issues, such as the availability of medications and the cost of medications that may be ignored in the office setting with patients with better insurance coverage. There has also been an attitudinal shift among the residents in that most of them now feel it is worthwhile to do this and good to be involved in the community. This may carry through into their own practices in the future and create a sense of broadened responsibility to the communities in which they work, rather than only to the patients in their offices. The project has met a need of community outreach for the hospital and the students. A future challenge is how to deal with the success of the project and expand with limited or no money. The hospital is exploring with the school some institutional ways to raise funds and also to obtain additional grant funding. Ideas of ways to raise money include doing active fund-raising events, such as a golf tournament and a ball in which the profits are directed to community involvement efforts of the hospital, with a special focus on the school activities. Some of the employee fund-raising in the hospital may also focus on this. The school district and hospital are still considering whether it might be possible for them to apply for some new special state funding linked to tobacco control funds. For one additional year, the principal was able to obtain a Neighborhood Fight Back grant to help provide funds through the city of Phoenix. The school uses this to help with supplies and other things for which the Flinn money was used in the first 2 years of the project. The pharmacy effort will be supported partially by these funds.

The hospital has indicated that it is quite committed to this project (more than to many of its other outreach efforts) and that unless the central mission of the hospital and the residency program changes drastically, it expects the program to continue. The hospital has included this project in its new strategic plan that starts in September and has also included trying to expand to another school in the near future. The director of the residency program has described the project as "the showpiece of community involvement for the hospital."

This has become a stable, well-accepted project in which the partnership between the hospital and the people in the school and the district is strengthening over time. One unique aspect of this project is that the direct providers are themselves residents and are still receiving educational benefits from providing services to children within a school setting. The gain the hospital receives for the residents in training helps to build the hospital's commitment to continuing the project and is an important reason why this project is likely to continue in its present form for many years. The clinic is well accepted by parents and teachers, and one indication of this is the growth in use of the clinic in the second year. The time of the residents is now probably as busy with patients as is feasible. This project is an affordable, lower-cost model that has used Flinn funds for the purchase of equipment and supplies but is sustainable without a large amount of grant funds.

The presence of a committed administrator in the school was critical to the initial forming of the partnership, and the principal has continued to look for other sources of funding to help with medications. Thus, the partnership between an interested school, a willing school nurse (who has been very positive at all stages about the project), and a hospital with a residency program has proven to be a sustainable and affordable model, even though the range of services provided is modest. The services are modest, given that the school-based clinic is open only one morning per week and that, in the first year, medications were less available. Lab services and x-rays continue to be less available than in some of the projects that have a more comprehensive model of care. Yet children at the school have clearly benefitted, the project is viewed within the district as enough of a success that the district would be happy to see an expansion to cover a second school, and the model is sustainable at minimal cost. Thus, this project indicates how modest goals and a less comprehensive approach may at times lead to a sustainable and successful project.

Phoenix 3

Phoenix 3 was one of the group of Flinn Foundation projects funded in the second year. This project was awarded a 2-year grant from August 1994 through August 1996. It was started at the initiative of the school district in cooperation with a federally funded health clinic that had been a rural health clinic as the medical partner. Unlike the other Phoenix projects located in the city, this project is located in a rural community adjoining Maricopa County, the county in which Phoenix is located. The community is undergoing change from a rural economy to a transitory tourist-based economy, and perhaps eventually a suburban economy. Now many of the parents of children in the school are employed in jobs with minimum hourly wages and often great seasonal fluctuation in hours worked. The unemployment rate in 1989 was over 10%. The initial goal was to create a school-based clinic in one school, staffed with a family nurse practitioner from the clinic. The school district wished to charge a fee of about $80 for one child per semester for parents who committed to the school-based clinic as a source of care. The clinic agreed with this goal and wanted the clinic to be owned by the school district and thus have the license issued to the school district.

This is a fairly poor community, with 43% of the community living below 200% of the federal poverty level and 17% living below the poverty level. In the school district, about 42% of children are receiving free or reduced lunch.

The role of the school district in this project was crucial. The school district initially formed a health and wellness committee to talk about health care needs.

A needs assessment of the district was conducted. The committee recommendation was for a comprehensive model (although operating only 3 days a week) that would start with a school-based clinic at the elementary level and expand to include at least one dental exam a year and would be integrated with an existing program in the district of outreach that currently provides clothing, food, funds for utilities, and other social service help to 485 families.

The clinic did not begin operation as quickly as planned. Both delays in licensing and changes in personnel at the clinic led to delays in opening. No quantitative operational data were collected. The focus of the project was on opening of the clinic and on plans to continue the clinic after grant funds were no longer available.

This project was classified as a broader model because of the goals of the school district and the presence in the district of a project that tries to help low-income families with basic needs and emergencies. The program is administered by a district employee who works in the community and arranges donations of clothing, household items, food, and money and uses these to help pay rent, medical care, and medicines for needy families. Before the creation of the clinic, this office worked with local dentists and eye doctors to obtain free or discounted care.

This project encountered a number of special problems, including limitations with its health partner. The clinic did not view this as a long-term project, since its major facility was near the school district — only a small satellite clinic was. Though willing to help the school district begin the project, the health partner was not committed to a long-term role. To complicate matters, the clinic's nurse practitioner in this location resigned in December 1994, making it difficult for the clinic to send a provider into the school once the license was obtained. While trying to begin operations, the clinic helped the school district to obtain a nurse practitioner from a hospital in the area for the next fall.

The clinic did open that next fall with a provider through the hospital who was working with a different school-based clinic in another nearby school district. Unlike many of the other projects, the school district does hold the license for this clinic. They started the year with a fee for use of the clinic of $80 per semester per child, but enrollment was slow. The clinic changed its model to charging $5 dollars a visit on a fee-for- service basis.

As the program currently operates, parents at all four elementary schools and the middle school in the district can sign up with the project, and clinics are held 2 days a week. The social services project already operating in the district helps to coordinate transportation between schools because on-site services are available only at one school.

Issues of referral sources and follow-up in the summer remain. The clinic closes in the summer, and referrals for most other types of care (eye, dental needs) will continue to be handled through the existing social services project. Dental services are especially important. In the clinic's early operation, the nurse practitioner found that almost every child had some dental problems, but the hospital provided no backup in this area. Access to funds for medications is also a continuing issue.

Attention has focused on beginning and sustaining the clinic and winning the support of parents and teachers in the district so that the clinic is utilized to its full extent. The lack of a supportive and committed health partner limits the potential of this project and underscores the important role that a committed health partner may play in a successful school-based clinic.

Phoenix 4

Phoenix 4 is using a different model from any of the other school projects, one that in the table in the earlier section was described as a case management model. The school views itself as developing a health partnership with the community (in this case, parents of children at the school) and with a local hospital to help provide a continuum of health care services.

The project was initially a collaboration between a hospital and one particular elementary school and now is a partnership with the district. Initially, it was proposed for only 13 months. Its broad goals included ensuring that its families had access to a comprehensive continuum of services. A project focusing on developing a specific preliminary action plan had already been funded by the department of health service, division of maternal and child health in the state. More specific plans with the new funds were to restructure the role of the school nurse and the provision of daily routine nursing care in the school. The school nurse role would be expanded to provide case management to students and outreach and education to parents.

Case management is a concept receiving much discussion in the health care system today. It usually refers to helping a person with a health problem (the case) figure out how to have his or her health care problem managed through the different types of providers in the health care system. The model includes the concept of a continuum of care. Good case management should help deal with a problem from its initial occurrence as a minor outpatient issue to a hospitalization episode to finding continuing care if a person needs that. The concept is discussed the most in the context of care for the elderly and hospital discharge planning, and, more recently, within health maintenance organizations. Within a school setting, the application of the model is different from that of a typical school clinic model. In Phoenix 4, the model included having the school nurse become involved the first time a child reported a health problem and having the nurse determine if more care was needed. If more care was needed, the nurse would contact the parent, determine health insurance coverage, and then follow different steps to try to have the child taken care of, depending on the health insurance situation. If the child had private health insurance (very few actually did at the school) or was currently enrolled in an AHCCCS plan, the school nurse served as a case manager and tried to ensure that the child went to the appropriate provider. If transportation was an issue, the school would help. An important aspect of the case model as developed by the school was helping those on AHCCCS to be seen by their provider. The nurse was familiar with a number of anecdotal situations in which mothers of children were unable to have children seen in reasonable amounts of time for acute care problems. For example, the mother of a child with an ear infection was not able to receive a doctor visit within 2 weeks. In fact, it was these types of anecdotes that led the school to develop a case management model. The model assumed that the school nurse (being middle class, fluent in English, and more able to manipulate bureaucracies, as well as knowledgeable of how to threaten or actually report the plan to the overall administration of AHCCCS) would be able to help obtain timely visits for sick children, even when mothers had not been able to obtain such visits. If no insurance was available, one option was to have the child seen by the nurse practitioner at the school-based clinic or referred to the nurse practitioner at the pediatric clinic of the hospital partner. If children were judged AHCCCS eligible, the nurse practitioner would help with the immediate problem, but then the case manager would help the family become enrolled in AHCCCS.

The school served about 850 children in Grades K through 6. There was about a 50% turnover in the school population each year. The demographics of the school were about 38% Hispanic. The principal estimated that about 70% of those students spoke only Spanish in the home. The school had a high Native American enrollment (22%), with other major groups being Anglo white (33%) and African Americans (5%). About 91% of the students were eligible for free and reduced lunch. About half of the school students were covered by AHCCCS, and about 23% had no health care coverage. One example of the unmet need for care of children in this school was that during a speech, hearing, and language screening of kindergartners, 61% of children were found to have some degree of hearing loss and 41% to have a middle-ear problem.

The school had children with many serious social and health problems and had had a substantial number of children referred to behavioral services over the previous few years. They had seven children diagnosed with fetal alcohol syndrome.

For the initial year, the grant funds were used to hire a health aide, who provided daily routine health care for the school children. This allowed the nurse practitioner to use most of her time as a case manager. In addition, a nurse practitioner from the hospital made daily visits.

The role of the hospital partner changed over the 2 years. By the end of the 2 years, the school had a goal of providing more comprehensive services linking social and health and educational needs, and the school obtained some funding from the health department. The social worker for the district was pivotal, along with the hospital, whose commitment increased as the project developed. This project became attractive as a way for the hospital to become involved in health care problems of the urban poor on a small scale. Their initial thoughts had been to develop a single school-based clinic, but as the partnership was put together, the school personnel were found to already have some ideas about what they felt would be the best model.

As the school and hospital personnel talked together, the case management model became clearer as one in which the hospital would serve as backup both for the school-based clinic services and for more serious health care needs of the children. The willingness of the nurse practitioner at the clinic to share her time with the hospital became important in the project. On average, the nurse practitioner came to the school three times a week, generally at lunch, although sometimes she stopped by in the morning. Generally, she saw two to four students at the clinic. One issue for the project was that the nurse practitioner was spending (based on her own estimates) 2 hours a day on the project, one as her lunch hour and one donated from the hospital. The hospital management was concerned her ability to maintain this enthusiasm and the potential for burnout. In this project, unlike some other projects in which the nurse practitioner sees all children who present with a problem, the nurse practitioner saw only children without health insurance or with such acute health care problems that they could not wait to be put on AHCCCS. When children were already on AHCCCS, case management was used to have them seen by the AHCCCS provider. During the first year, 14,058 visits to the school nurses's office occurred. Of these, 1,925 involved receiving some case management by the school nurse. In the first half of the next school year, the project continued to serve about 990 children for case management out of about 8,000 visits to the school nurse's office. The nurse practitioner provided care to 75 children, and 10 were referred for extended care to the hospital pediatric ambulatory clinic.

Both the social worker and the school nurse viewed this partnership as part of a larger effort of connecting the school as an institution (and the children and their families) to other community institutions. The social worker had become very concerned about unmet needs of many types in the community (food, clothing, medical) and was convinced that these had an impact on the education of the children. The social worker (who worked for the school district, not just the school) was very committed to expanding social services in the district and creatively used internships to do this. She viewed this school as the most appropriate school in the district to begin a health-related project because of the commitment and enthusiasm of the school nurse and her past background as a public health nurse. She was interested in trying to apply what she saw as a broadened public health model to school nursing. She also wanted to become involved in giving parents health education and teaching them when and how to use the health care system to maintain their child's health and ability to learn in the school.

By the end of the first year, some positive spin-offs from the initial project had occurred. The hospital obtained a grant from its corporate offices to provide dental care for children at the school. Additional funding was obtained through United Way so that the health aide would continue at the school, allowing the school nurse to function as a case manager. The school started a Family Resource Center as part of being a Chapter 1 school and used this to make food available and provide some English and parenting classes to parents. By the end of the next year, a grant from a local corporation was obtained that ensured continued funds for the project for 3 more years, along with funds for some expansion of services throughout the school district.

This model must be evaluated quite differently from the more traditional school-based clinic model. Only a few children (about 20 a month) are being seen by the nurse practitioner at the clinic. The major contact with the schoolchildren, their parents, and the community is the case management efforts of the school nurse. The school has some limited data to indicate that attendance is better from children who have seen the nurse practitioner in the past year as compared to the previous year. Thus, the school is convinced that the project has helped children at the school. The model continues to evolve.

By the third year of operation of the project, the role of the school nurse had begun to change. She was no longer the provider at her school but worked with the district headquarters, as did the social worker. The private corporate funds were used to expand the case management model to the total district. One more on-site clinic was licensed at another elementary school. Part of the corporate grant funds was used to hire three health home school liaisons (most of whom had a background at the bachelor's level in social work) who would be the people to help parents become AHCCCS eligible, help them to obtain appointments with their doctors, and possibly even accompany them to the visit and help to interpret the statements of the health care provider to them. The person who was the school nurse originally at the first school now functions as the health care expert on the project; she receives all of the referrals and then contacts the home school liaisons.

One limitation is that in the initial years the nurse practitioner continued, in essence, to donate her lunch time for many days. As the model gradually expands to other schools in this district, it is unclear whether these schools will transport children to the on-site clinics or whether the hospital will make another practitioner available, with a certain number of hours per week. This person would also have to donate some of his or her own free time. The hospital administrator dealing with the project did say that the hospital might budget a salary for a nurse practitioner to the project that would be spread across several nurse practitioners. Thus, the issue of the linkage between the hospital, the nurse practitioner, and the school was not totally clear.

The project placed great emphasis on helping all children to find a medical home. The project helped those not AHCCCS eligible to become registered at the hospital pediatric ambulatory clinic, at which fees were generally $15 a month to cover the care of all the children in the family if the family was poor but not AHCCCS eligible. In the early project years, the the numbers did not overwhelm the clinic but helped to demonstrate the need for the continuation of the clinic as a charity-based service of the hospital.

The school district has reactivated its community foundation so that it can receive donations. It is trying to work with more local businesses and has managed to arrange for charity events to raise funds for the foundation, although it is doubtful that these funds alone will ever be enough to maintain the project.

Other activities the project has explored are receiving some AHCCCS funds or state tobacco funds. The district is convinced that the case management model is a leaner model to provide services for children than a major school-based clinic effort. The district has modified its case management model to use BSW social workers for much of the actual case management work. Grant funds will also pay for a half-time data clerk so that quantitative data will be available in the future. The project is also hiring a half-time clerk to aid in assorted tasks.

This project has clearly been successful initially. The project is refining its case management model, which is an interesting alternative to more typical school-based clinics and may well be less expensive than many other approaches. For other districts to adopt this model, some funding for case management would be required. The project must obtain its own funds through grants. It is clear that the project would not have succeeded in this district without a very committed nurse and social worker. Not all districts have social workers, and this model does not appear feasible without these kinds of resources.

In addition, the nurse practitioner's willingness to donate her time made the project possible. The availability of a backup clinic was also critical. If these had not been available, it is less clear what the case management model could have accomplished. It could have helped to obtain care for AHCCCS children but not to provide a medical home or backup for "notch group" children and other children not eligible for AHCCCS (such as children of undocumented parents). Thus, despite the substantial success of the project at this point and its innovative application of an interesting model, the model may not be exportable to other school districts. Having a good health care partner is essential to success, as is having unusually committed and motivated nursing and social work personnel.

Southern Arizona 2

This project was a joint effort between a school district outside the major Tucson metropolitan area in southern Arizona and an outpatient health center in that community that receives federal funds as part of the community health centers and has an obligation to have services available on a sliding-scale basis. All the other Tucson projects became part of one model and are discussed after this project. Unlike the other Arizona projects discussed so far, this project was part of a high school. Providing services in a high school can generate a higher level of controversy in the community because the issue of reproductive health services can become an issue of concern. This did happen, and the project had one of the rockier starts, with controversy about lack of initial notification provided to the school board.

Some background on this community is helpful. The location of the community near the Mexico border creates special issues, both of a complicated economy and of a different population mix (predominantly Mexican American). At the time the project began, the town's economy was good, but by the end of the

Flinn funding portion, the economy of the town was suffering because of the devaluation of the Mexican peso and the weakness of the Mexican economy. This had changed the overall atmosphere within the school from one of optimism about the future of the town to one of great concern about the future.

The high school itself had about 1,800 students, with a mobile population and fairly high dropout rate, especially among males. Estimates were that about 75% of students qualified for free or reduced lunch and Chapter 1 services. The school was about 95% Hispanic.

The initial proposal was a joint effort of the school district and the clinic. It had two overall goals: to increase students' access to comprehensive health care and to improve the overall health, well-being, and educational performance of adolescents. Included as part of this was the creation of a peer health counselors program to educate students on issues related to drug use, teen pregnancy, and self-help behaviors and to assist teens to network with needed mental health and social services in the community. The initial proposal was for a clinic that would be staffed 8 hours a week.

This project was categorized as "limited" because of its focus on less extensive school-based services, which continued as the project developed. Some initial goals, as listed above, were more comprehensive, especially the inclusion of a peer counseling program and some parent and staff training, but few of these were actually accomplished. The project was also categorized as having equal participation by the health care partner and the school district, especially in its planning stages and first year.

This project had a shakier beginning than some of the others because after the funding award was announced by the Flinn Foundation, it became clear that the school board had not been appropriately notified about the proposal and had not really agreed to allow the proposal to begin. Although the clinic had worked with the school district, although the head of school nursing had notified and received the permission of the principal of the school, and although the superintendent of the school district had been notified and had approved of the project, the board had never been notified. Thus, much of the beginning time of the grant focused on the question of whether the school board would formally approve the proposal. This lack of explicit agreement by the school board allowed opposition to occur, based both on fears about a clinic in the high school and the types of services it might offer and on some conflict within the community between private practitioners and those who practiced medicine at the clinic. Eventually, the board approved the project.

After that, a community advisory board had to be formed that represented most interests in the community. As formed, the board had three members appointed by the school board and three by the clinic, with one of those being a parent of a high-school-aged child, one a physician from the clinic, and one a member of the board of the clinic. As a result of all this discussion, some initial plans for the project were changed, and most were delayed. Initially, part of the plan was for the school district to actually run the clinic and for part of the grant funds to support nursing staff relief in the district. The final decision after the project was approved by the board was that, for purposes of controlling liability and appropriateness, the clinic would provide a formal lease arrangement and would "own" the clinic and the license, only leasing space from the school district.

As with many of the projects, the obtaining of the license for the clinic was itself a hurdle, in this case compounded first by lengthy negotiations over a lease. In addition, the initial model for operating the clinic was to staff with volunteers, both from the clinic and from private practice. Volunteers served at the school clinic in addition to their regular clinical time seeing patients. The initial volunteer list was substantial and included both nurse practitioners and physicians from the health center and the community. As with other projects, but exacerbated in this case by the delays due to the need for school board approval, the clinic was able to open for less than a month of the first year of the project. This became a small test run for the next year.

The clinic reopened at the beginning of the 1994-95 school year, still operating with volunteers mostly from the clinic, although one physician and one nurse practitioner from the community also volunteered. It was open only 1 day a week, on Wednesday, for 4 hours (rather than 8 as initially proposed). It reported 178 encounters, primarily with high school students, although there were nine visits by school staff members. Women were responsible for 51.7% of the encounters and men for 48.3%. The maximum number of encounters for any one person was five. Only three other individuals were seen more than twice, and a total of 141 different individuals were seen. Depending on how one considers these data, they could reveal a strength or weakness of the project. Many different students were being seen (a strength), but very few individuals returned after the initial visit. It is not clear if this indicates a "silent" dissatisfaction with the services of the clinic or the specific provider seen (who for any one student was likely to have been a different person from the one seen by another student, given that multiple providers were in the clinic over the year). It also may imply that students were using the clinic for short-term acute problems. The most commonly reported reasons for visits for the clinic were colds, followed by physicals, and then the "other" category, with the injury and skin categories also fairly large. Less than 4% of visits were for pregnancy concerns, a low figure in a school district with a substantial number of teenage pregnancies reported each year. This low figure may indicate that students were unwilling to use the clinic for these types of problems. At least two different interpretations are possible. One is that, perhaps due to the many different providers, students did not feel confident and were unwilling to trust the clinic. Another suggestion, pointed out by some of the personnel at the school, is that because the clinic is in the school and other students can tell when a student goes there (or might be able to), there could be a sensitivity about others noting a student going to the clinic when he or she appears well.

During the fall semester of 1994, an administrative change in the project occurred. The first administrator of the project left the clinic, leaving the school district representative, the head of nursing, more important for the success of the project. Despite the rough start, many operational aspects of the clinic worked smoothly. Consent forms were filled out at the time of enrollment by ninth-grade parents, and three fourths of the way through the 1994-95 school year, the school had consent forms from about 30% of students. The school nurse referred patients to the clinic, and specific times of operation were announced through the morning bulletin 2 days before the clinic.

One problem was the limited amount of time the clinic could be open and thus the inability to build a constituency for the clinic. Also, there was some disagreement on what the real goals of the school clinic should be from the perspective of school personnel versus the providers. The providers saw the clinic more as a "sickness" clinic to deal with acute health care needs. The school personnel wanted the clinic to have a broader "wellness" focus that would include educating high school students about health and about how to use the health care system wisely as they became adults. As long as volunteers were contributing time and different people staffed the clinic not only from week to week but even from month to month, it was difficult to reconcile these differing images of the clinic and its goals.

Over the year of full operation, these issues surfaced even more clearly. School personnel very much wanted to have the clinic staffed for half of each school day (an increase from the initial proposal). As the year progressed, the clinic was generally only staffed one half-day a week, and which day of the week that was varied depending on the times that the health care providers had available. Use of the clinic was fairly low. Whereas on some days providers might see eight or more students a morning, on other days they might see only two or three. Through March of the first year of full operation, the most patients seen on any one day was nine and the least was two. Although school officials were convinced that if students knew the clinic was open each morning or each afternoon, they would be more likely to use it, other issues included trust. Teenagers are unlikely to turn to an unknown and not-trusted provider for health concerns of a private and potentially embarrassing nature.

Whether the clinic would sporadically provide a few health services or whether it would be a more comprehensive wellness center open for more hours remained an issue. The project as proposed in the grant to the Flinn Foundation did include mental health, wellness, and educational activities, but these did not materialize. Whether all school personnel wanted the broader model was unclear. The volunteer providers did not share a vision of mental health and emotional problems as problems that they wanted to treat in this setting.

One peer counseling activity was planned at the beginning of the year with eight students. Two dropped out due to class schedules, and an additional two were dropped due to lack of attendance. Over the year, five to six students actively participated in most sessions.

There were some positive spin-offs from the creation of the clinic. Other agencies in the community are now viewing the school district and the high school as a place from which to deliver services, and the school has been in contact with some other types of community agencies about offering services at the school site.

Stable future funding remains a major issue. Though the school district has tried working with the other major health provider in town, most options that would provide a nurse practitioner for half a day require grant money.

Despite the early political issues, political support for the school-based clinic now appears quite solid. A new community board is in place and has been working on issues productively. The school board is quite comfortable now with the clinic and supportive of expanded hours of operation if they can be supported without school district funds. Other major political actors in the community are also satisfied with the clinic.

Although this clinic has been a modest effort in terms of numbers of hours open, range of services provided, and numbers of students served, one mark of its success up to this point is that it has remained functioning after the Flinn grants funds were exhausted. Though both clinic personnel and school health and administrative personnel believe that the clinic could be more successful and more useful to students and their parents if it were open more regularly, this is unlikely with volunteer labor.

In general, arrangements of volunteered time are difficult to maintain unless both parties are receiving substantial value from the arrangement (as in the Phoenix 2 project). In this community, the clinic really gains little from the arrangement except the potential for attracting new patients and good will in the community. Because the physicians and nurse practitioners donate part of their time not designated for patient care, they need to receive some benefit from giving up this time. Initially, some volunteers hoped to gain more experience with adolescents, but the low use rates in the clinic have frustrated them. Also, the school is happy using the school-based clinic for sports physicals, but the health care practitioners do not see this as an appropriate use of their time. The initial support of an advocate from within the school district (the director of school nursing) was quite important, and she has continued to be a spokesperson for the project and to impart to the principal and clinic personnel her vision of the role of the school-based clinic in the future.

The declining economy of the town may make survival of the school-based clinic even more difficult if state revenues are not obtained. The option of soliciting funds from local businesses and using donations to continue to operate does not seem likely to succeed in this community at this point. Interestingly, the early political problems caused by the lack of school board approval initially, has not resurfaced. In fact, political support for the program and its expansion now is strong, and continued operation is much more a question of money and time commitment than an issue of any community or political opposition.

Southern Arizona 1, 3, and 4

This is the most complicated project, partially because it began as three separate projects and eventually merged into one. Southern Arizona 1 was the first project and involved collaboration between the major school district in the area and a federally funded health clinic to establish a school-based health clinic at a middle school. The second and third project involved collaboration between the same school district as in Southern Arizona 1 and several others; Southern Arizona 3 also involved a federally related health clinic, and Southern Arizona 4 involved a university-affiliated group of physicians. Southern Arizona 3 started during the second year of the initial grants, as did Southern Arizona 4, although its clinics did not open until January 1995.

All three of these projects are now clearly part of one larger effort under a new name of Family Resource and Wellness Centers (FRWCs), a broader model that the projects in this area have adopted. This project has grown in complexity over the years because not only are the health clinics one portion of a broader model but a number of different coalitions have been formed. One coalition is among the different school districts that participate in the FRWC model. Another was formed by the end of the Flinn Foundation involvement with the projects.

The beginnings of the first project were somewhat different from those of the two projects added the next year, and each project has unique aspects. This section will first provide some background on each project and the overall FRWC model and then discuss each project separately.

Clearly, the overall FRWC approach, in which the school-based or related health clinic is one component, represents an "expansive" model (although in its original proposal, this applied least to Southern Arizona 1). As for the roles of the two partners, the two newer projects (Southern Arizona 3 and 4) are definitely examples of a more important role for the school district, for by then the FRWC model and an overall approach to its implementation were further developed than had been true 9 to 12 months earlier. In the Southern Arizona 1 project, initial roles were more equal for the two partners. It was the health clinic that first decided to apply for funds from the foundation, and only because of success in obtaining those funds did the clinic learn more about the overall approach. As the clinic was first set up (and with the agreement of the clinic and the administrator of the school at which the clinic was located), its services were limited to the children in the school and its nearby schools, not the total community.

The Southern Arizona 1 project was first and was a joint venture between two local health care corporations, a federally funded health center, and a school district. The project's initial goals were to pilot and plan school-based health services for Head Start, elementary, and middle-school-age children. Specific aims of the project were to improve physical and emotional health of the students, to improve student and family knowledge of preventive health practices, to improve health practices, to increase early detection and treatment of acute and chronic illness, and to reduce school absences and lost work time due to child illness.

Southern Arizona 3 included two school districts, the one from Southern Arizona 1 and another local school district. It was a project begun in the second year but was part of a broadened model of how to implement school clinics. By the beginning of the 1994-95 school year, the nurse practitioner was able to begin holding clinics in both projected locations. The main goals of this project were to fit within the broader FRWC model, and the two clinics established were located somewhat apart from any specific school. In one case, a family resource center without health care services had already been open for a year, located in a portion of a no longer operative old school near a new school building. The health clinic was also located in the old school building. In the second district involved with this project, both the health clinic and family resource center were located in an old school building that was now being used for a variety of adult education programs and alternative high school programs.

Southern Arizona 4 project also began in the second year of the Flinn projects. This project involved a university medical school as the main health partner, an HMO, and a physician group along with two local school districts. The project wanted to pilot-test three school-based clinics within the FRWC model: two located at elementary schools and one in a high school. The two goals were to develop a long-term plan to comprehensively serve students in targeted high-risk sections of the metropolitan area and to demonstrate the effectiveness of school-based services to promote health and prevent illness. At one site, there was to be special coordination and work with a demonstration project with the local Council on Aging. In the initial proposal, health services would be provided by a family nurse practitioner for two mornings a week at one of the elementary schools and the high school and one morning a week at the other elementary school. This project included a training component for family medicine residents, medical students, and nurse practitioner students. The FRWC approach was developed as a collaborative effort between four of the metropolitan school districts in the county, the major city in the county, the county government, the Arizona State Department of Economic Security, and various other parental, governmental, educational, and community agencies. These groups are engaged in a long-term effort to effect institutional change, guarantee ongoing cooperation, and develop an effective school-linked service delivery system for children and families. The effort began in the fall of 1992 when members of the four school boards initiated a meeting with the mayor to discuss what school districts could do to better address needs of students and families. From this first meeting, a School Districts' Action Task Force was formed with several areas of priority: safety, FRWCs, expanded use of schools for parks, recreation, youth programs and library services, child care, and miscellaneous services such as tutoring, counseling, mediation, improved transportation, and enriched educational opportunities. The focus of the 1992-93 and 1993-94 school years was the development and implementation of 12 to 13 FRWC sites in neighborhoods with the highest problems, with 10 more FRWC sites to be added in 1994-95. Thus, the health component was one specified interest, although not a major effort in the first 2 years. The Flinn Foundation provided funds that allowed several health projects to start, although this was not coordinated through the overall FRWCs.

Southern Arizona 1 was the first operational school-based health clinic in the area. It began with a more traditional model of a school-based clinic rather than the overall approach of the FRWC model. The initial plan was to staff a clinic at the middle school with a pediatric nurse practitioner (PNP), aided by an LPN. She would see children from the middle school and three nearby elementary schools. Children were to be referred to the clinic by the school nurses, classroom teachers, or principals. On the basis of the original proposal, the school district would provide the space and utilities, and the clinic would provide the PNP and supplies through the grant. The first change required for the clinic was to partially adapt the broader goals of the FRWC sites. Although the clinic had not planned this project in concert with the overall FRWC sites, it had worked with the major school district before on teen clinics. Clinic personnel felt that schools were an important site to reach youth, and they wanted to gain more experience working with schools. That is why they applied initially for Flinn funding.

At the school site, the principal was less enthusiastic than some about his school as a site for the clinic. He did hope that the clinic might increase the community's connection to the school, for the school then operated as a magnet school, mostly serving middle-school-age children living outside the neighborhood. One of the principal's major concerns was space. He preferred the clinic to operate from a portable building located on the school grounds because of limited space in the nurse's office, but the clinic opened initially in the nurse's office. The opening was exciting but confusing. More clients spoke only Spanish than expected. Because the PNP had only limited Spanish skills, this meant that the head of the FRWC, a former social worker with the school district, had to interpret. An LPN was not hired for the spring. The clinic experienced many no-shows and averaged only three patients a day, partially due to limited contact between the school nurse and the clinic and thus few referrals from the school itself. One explanation for this is that the middle school was a magnet school, and a substantial proportion of the population of the school was more affluent than the neighborhood. In this project, most patients at the encounters were Hispanic (75.3%). Boys were seen in 53.3% of the visits, probably due to higher numbers of requests for sports physicals. After a year of operation, the clinic was still being held in the school. A trailer was on the school site but had to be refurbished to be appropriate for a clinic. Staffing was an issue because the PNP who initially staffed the clinic left her job at the health center. Because other clinics were now open, some children who needed care were transported to a different school clinic, an advantage of the FRWC coordination. The new person hired was a family nurse practitioner and thus was able to see adult patients from the community, not just children, and bilingual patients. Although utilization of the clinic improved, rates were still lower than those in the Southern Arizona 3 project clinics. Estimates were that about 80% of clients were on an AHCCCS plan, but used the clinic because of transportation difficulties in reaching their assigned provider. One positive aspect of the continued operation was that the principal, who initially feared having community personnel in the school because it might disrupt the educational process, decided that the clinic was not disruptive and was good for the community.

In contrast to the slow start of the Southern Arizona 1 project and the continued slow rate of accumulation of patients, the Southern Arizona 3 project started quickly in the 1994-95 school year and began seeing large numbers of patients. A nurse practitioner at this site split her time between two clinics. She saw many patients, but with little help, so she could complete only minimally required clinical records. The two clinics that were part of this project were more closely integrated with the FRWC approach and were located nearer to those services. The community acceptance of these sites was high, with the nurse practitioner seeing 16 to 18 patients a day, a large number. This practitioner spoke Spanish, a major asset in this community. The Southern Arizona 3 project reported the largest number of encounters, a total of 1,462 in its first 9 months of operation. Because the clinic was open to the community, 51.7% of encounters were for those over age 14, and 48.3% for those under age 14. The age category with the most visits was the aged 20 to 40 category (21.5%). Most visits were for illness (41.1%) and "other" (34.5%) categories, followed by injury (9%) and counseling (7.3%). The identified problems varied, with the most common being sport physicals (18.6%) and cold-related problems (18.4%). The nurse practitioner also received about 12 to 15 phone calls a week from nurses at nearby schools who had heard about the clinic. One concern in this project is the very high workload of the nurse practitioner with no administrative or clinical relief.

One reason for success of this project initially was that it started later, after the model had been thought through more and after the FRWC services were available at those sites. Community people trusted the facility overall and were willing to try the health care available. Another reason was the nurse practitioner herself, who took control of the project and bought supplies and helped to arrange referral sources for children though her own personal networks. She was well liked by community residents, leading to increased use of the clinic.

Southern Arizona 4 was started as an FRWC site, and one of the goals of the affiliated university was training. Unfortunate events hindered this project from the beginning. The high school at which one clinic was planned had a fire in the fall, and thus all spare space that had been set aside for the clinic had to be used for classroom space, delaying the opening of that clinic. Further, obtaining licenses was slow. Once the clinics did open, the nurse practitioner was seeing, on average, 10 to 12 patients a session and was going to each elementary school twice a week for half a day. The nurse practitioner with this project was quite experienced and had worked with similar types of clinics in other states. She believed that through the community contacts of the FRWC personnel and by conducting inservices with the teachers to make them aware of the range of services that the clinic could provide, she could quickly see an appropriate number of clients per session at the elementary schools. The Southern Arizona 4 project reported 630 encounters in about 5 months. Ages of patients in this site were widely distributed, with 27.9% of patients under the age of 7, 35% ranging from age 7 to 11 years, and 37.1% over the age of 12. Most visits to the Southern

Arizona 4 project clinics were for illness or well-child visits. The major identified health problems were earache (20.6%), colds (19%), and regular or sports physicals (19%). Medication was the most common treatment, used in 48.4% of all encounters.

The high school clinic never opened during the 1994-95 school year because of the fire. There were also some questions about being able to quickly attract high school students into the facility, based mostly on the reluctance of high school students to trust new facilities and providers. The nurse practitioner at this project was enthusiastic about working with teenagers at this site, as all of the other clinics in this project were connected to schools with younger students.

By the end of the 1994-95 school year, the major issue for all the projects was whether they would be functioning by the next fall and whether they would each continue to work somewhat separately with their own health care partners or whether the model would be more centrally coordinated. One idea in place by May 1995 was that a new 501C corporation would be established that dealt only with the health aspect of the projects and that a separate 501C corporation would handle the non-medical aspects of the FRWC model. One solution was possible federal funding, and a $200,000 grant was submitted in the spring but was not funded. A Kellogg grant was also under discussion. The major prospects for continued funding of the health care centers were to form a coalition of health care providers and possibly to charge fees for some services. Obtaining funding from AHCCCS was another possibility to keep the six planned and operational sites open. The forming of a new corporation would provide lease agreements with each district and one health care provider who obtained licenses for all the clinics to simplify coordination. Clinics remained open, although with breaks in service delivery over the summer and part of the fall. Of the five clinics that were initially opened through these three projects, three remained open over most of the summer and fall. The other two opened or reopened in the spring of 1996. A new group, the 501-C, was formed to run the health partnership and remains in operation. The new organization has a board of directors and an executive director (one of the board members from the major school district) and a series of three different sets of contracts: one for clinical services with several clinics and hospitals, one with the school districts, and one for billing services with one of the clinics. Overall, eight health centers were in operation by April 1995 and serve the major needy areas of the county. Plans are underway to try to bill AHCCCS for some services, and a few clinics have instituted a $5 copayment.

These three Southern Arizona projects were the most ambitious of all the projects. Some small lessons are clear. It is better to hire family nurse practitioners than PNPs, especially if the goal is to have a clinic for both adults in the community and the children in the school. Full-time providers work better than part-time ones who also have other clinical responsibilities. In this part of the state, the nurse practitioner must be able to communicate with parents or older patients in Spanish.

Although the overall approach is impressive, this is one of the most expensive models and, for that reason alone, is more susceptible to failure if funds become tighter. Grant funds from various sources, such as health providers and United Way, are currently being used. The strength of the project at this point is that existing clinics are continuing operation and new ones are being added. The amount of services that these clinics are providing is substantial, and the organization of their services is strong. Future success depends on further rationalizing the administrative processes in terms of overall leadership of the project, continuing to find funding, and hiring good, personable, and committed nurse practitioners for the clinics as they open.

STATE EFFORTS IN ARIZONA IN 1997

Most of this chapter has discussed recent projects funded by a local foundation grant, but some school-based and school-linked centers in Arizona were started as early as 1988 (although the first one did not provide medical care). As the model has developed in Arizona, the Arizona Department of Health Services now tracks what it labels "community-based centers," which include school-based or school-linked centers (Arizona Department of Health Services, 1997). Arizona's model of community-based centers is premised on the system development concept. Self-defined communities will develop services based on local needs. Thus, not all of the centers will provide direct medical care services, and some will provide a broad range of services, whereas others may focus only on some health care services. Centers can be funded through community partnerships developed between schools, hospitals, community health centers, private foundations, philanthropic organizations, and tobacco tax special funding. Most centers have been established since 1994. As of the 1996-97 school year, centers were available in 12 of the 16 counties in the state, with 127 different sites in operation. Of these sites, 109 are school based, 14 are school linked, and 4 provide services from a mobile van. Most (77%) provide medical care. Behavioral health services are provided by 22%, and 41% provide social services of various types. In many ways, centers from one school district to the next share similarities (often in the type of provider, with nurse practitioners the most common type), but in other ways centers vary, from those that are open only 1 day a week (like some of the ones discussed in more detail earlier in this chapter) to those that are open every school day and much of the summer as well. Financing of the centers in Arizona remains a major concern.

In Arizona, many school-based health centers are now part of the School-Based Health Centers Program. This program is helping provide nurse practitioners and case coordinators for many schools. Funding varies from site to site. In the city of Phoenix, a number of hospitals and clinics are partners with various school districts, along with both national and local foundation funding. Some proceeds from the 40-cents-per-pack tobacco tax that was passed in 1994 are being allocated by the Arizona Department of Health Services to supplement primary care and some dental care services for schoolchildren. In 1996-97, about

$5 million was allocated to 52 school-based/school-linked programs, 15 clinic sites, and one mobile clinic (Ballantyne, 1997).

LESSONS LEARNED FROM THE ARIZONA PROJECTS

After this review of each of the Flinn-funded projects, one important question is what lessons can be learned. How successful were the different projects and models? Also, what specific advice could be given to new attempts to begin school-based clinics in other states? Some issues are important for the planning of projects and the initial implementation. Others are important operational issues that will continue as the clinics continue, and these issues will overlap. A third set of issues relates to how social and health services are made available to those in need in this society (thus, they concern more fundamental needs and solutions that are often beyond the resolution ability of any one school-based clinic). This set of issues is addressed in the concluding chapter of the book, as is the new federally-funded, state-administered child health insurance program. Implementation issues are an important aspect of evaluation of these projects. Some important lessons for both school districts and funding agencies are that these projects are more difficult to begin and take longer to move from the initial planning stage to the implementation stage of being fully open than the Flinn Foundation or most of the projects had realized. Almost none of the projects could meet the deadlines they had initially proposed. The only two that did were the projects in which the health care provider was already providing some services to a school in the district. Those projects were actually further along in planning and implementation than were the other projects. Thus, in any future planning and evaluation grant, a project needs to allow more start-up time, and the granting agency needs to give projects more time to obtain a license and work out contractual relationships. In Arizona, the state health department and a group of school-based clinics (including many of projects reviewed in detail in this chapter) have been meeting over the last 2 years and have developed a very specific, detailed manual that will help any new projects with applying for a license, understanding complex new regulations, and working out contractual leases between health care providers and school districts. Almost all of the projects experienced substantial delays due to such issues. Though understanding aspects of the process will help new clinics to begin operations more quickly, one lesson is that many of these steps take time and can only be rushed a small amount.

Another lesson from many of the projects is the need to develop more realistic budgets and staffing. These issues have been important for the implementation of many of the projects and will remain important in future years. If, for example, the nurse practitioner or other provider is expected to carry a full patient load and also to collect data to be used for evaluation for the project, there is a need for clerical support for the clinic, even if just from one of the secretaries in the school. In those projects in which the nurse practitioner was in a setting with little help of any type available (not in a school and thus without any nurse or clerk to help), having to handle data forms and clinical records became a very difficult (and not necessarily completed) burden. If data collection is desired in projects, the availability of a computer is critical. One project had included a computer in its initial budget, and because of that (and a nurse practitioner interested in data), it maintained the most complete data set.

During the first 1 to 2 years of operation, most projects became, in some ways, narrower than their aims. Though many of the grant proposals included a student education and even a parent or teacher education portion, most projects focused on having the clinic open, running smoothly, and obtaining enough support from parents, teachers, and students, in the case of high schools, so that the clinic was seeing a reasonable number of patients. Especially given the small amount of funds in most of these grants, ranging from about $25,000 in most cases to close to $50,000 in a few cases, there was neither enough time nor enough money to work on other issues, such as health education and prevention, along with the big issues of starting and operating the clinic. In the future, new projects should (at least initially) confine themselves to goals of providing clinical services or secure longer term grants and evaluate time frames. A longer time frame for the grants would have provided the opportunity to begin to look at outcomes, as well as the time to focus on issues beyond the immediate development of the clinic.

Another set of lessons concerns differences in types of schools and types of communities. Although nationally more of the school-based clinics have focused on adolescents, most of the projects reviewed here were in elementary or middle schools. Communities are often more supportive of programs for younger children, and those may be easier settings in which to begin clinics in a community. Controversies over what services are provided are not as common. Though keeping your community informed before you start is important advice for any project, it is more important for high schools, where the issues of whether the clinic will provide information and prescriptions for birth control and advice on human sexuality raise the level of concern among parents in the community. Of the projects reviewed here, the only one open in a high school during the first 2 years was the one with the most initial community conflict. Interestingly, the amount of that conflict at the beginning did not have a lasting impact on the project. After 2 years, the level of community support for that project did not appear to be a function of the initial controversy. One other special issue for high school clinics is that it is more difficult to convince teaching staff to be supportive. Teachers at the high school level are more focused on the academic subjects and often less involved with the details of the student's lives than elementary school teachers who see the student the entire day. This may be one reason (along with the generally good health of high school students) why teachers were less involved with the high school clinic. Related to this lesson is that schools are established bureaucracies and have established ways of doing things. The larger the district and the school, the more difficult it is to create change.

One lesson from many of these projects is the need for some sustainable source of funds for at least a half-time person. It is very difficult to sustain a project on all-volunteer effort. Only in cases in which both parties benefit (such as the residency program in one project) does it seem feasible to envision a project continuing for a number of years without a source of funds to help pay for the nurse practitioner or physician, whether by making an explicit change in the job description of an employee from a hospital or health clinic or by obtaining grant funds that allow the buyout of personnel time. Obtaining sustainable funds is one of the most critical issues. As previous literature has mentioned, few school-based clinics are able to survive on fees from students. In the most successful states, there have been state allocations either from the Maternal and Child Health Block Grant or from other state sources that provide a solid base of funding from year to year.

The last lesson for the opening of clinics relates to qualifications of the nurse practitioner or provider in the school. The person needs to be strong clinically but willing to try new things administratively, willing to work with computers to maintain data, and able to function independently much of the time. Thus, these clinics are not a good location for a new practitioner, for often the provider is working without easy access to clinical backup. In addition, depending on the population of the schools, rapport with the students and parents is helpful. In an increasingly diverse society, cultural sensitivity is very important. If many students or parents speak a different language (Spanish in the clinics reviewed in this chapter), the provider needs to be fluent in that language.

One important operational lesson is that some types of communities are places in which a clinic is more likely to succeed and obtain high utilization rates. The poorer the school is, the more isolated it is from the rest of the community (perhaps due to limited transportation), and the fewer people there are with health insurance, the more readily the clinic is accepted and the higher the utilization. Strong preexisting ties between the health care provider and the school and neighborhood, increase the chances for initial success of the project.

One issue for many projects is finding better sources of referrals for health care problems that are detected. Though all projects have some concerns about this, the issues are more serious for projects backed by smaller hospitals or community health clinics. What will happen if a serious health problem is detected, one that requires surgery and/or hospitalization? Only a few projects have had this happen so far, and they have been able to persuade a physician and hospital to deal with the problem. Only the school with the case management model and a connection with a pediatric ambulatory clinic through its hospital partner thinks that it knows how to handle such a situation. This may be a more serious issue in Arizona than in some other states because of the managed-care Medicaid model. In some states, once a very serious health problem is detected that is very expensive, it may be fairly easy for a child to qualify as medically needy, even though previously the child did not meet the qualification. This is less likely to occur in Arizona, given the operation of the AHCCCS program. Unless school-based clinics become more integrated with an overall care delivery system, such as AHCCCS, there will be no easy solutions. As other states move to managed-care Medicaid models, this will also be a limitation for them. Even more integration of services with AHCCCS will leave certain students without help, for at many of these schools some of the students are not AHCCCS eligible because the parents may be undocumented aliens. It does seem that, compared to community health clinics, a hospital is in a better position to provide backup resources (physicians, surgery, laboratory work). A hospital with a pediatric practice is in a stronger position to help with serious health problems than a hospital with a family practitioner emphasis.

Another major referral issue is the need for dental care. This was mentioned by almost all schools. Overall issues of how health and social services are provided in this country often ignore the serious but not life-threatening problems of both dental and eye care.

For projects to succeed, there needs to be strong support from both the health care provider and the school and its upper administration. Though different models of support can exist, the two projects with the more important role for the health provider seem the most sustainable without additional state support. As the state moves to provide some more stable revenues from special tax sources, more of the clinics may have a good chance to continue to exist. The impact of the new federal health funds may help, as well as continued availability of special state funds linked to a tobacco tax.

Although three of the Southern Arizona projects and two of the Phoenix projects have an image of the school of the future as more involved with the community and with the overall lives of children in the schools, not just with education, they have evolved different ways of developing health services within this basic framework. All three of these projects espouse the "full-service school" as their image of the best school for the future. But the Southern Arizona FRWC model places greater emphasis on extending the clinic beyond the school to the neighborhood. In contrast, the case management model of Phoenix 4 is more focused on the school and on obtaining services for those children (education, social services, health care, food services, etc.).

The most expansive initial models were the FRWCs. They have complicated plans for future funding, all of which have not yet been realized. If they work, the projects will continue and be a major success. In contrast, the case management model clinic already operates within a school district with more commitment to social services than in some other places. As currently developed, this model also requires substantial funds (unless the school district assumes the funding of a health aide at some schools along with a school nurse so that the school nurse could can continue as a case manager), which the school district has obtained for the next several years through grants, but which has not been incorporated into the regular district budget. The success of case management is being copied in some projects. If there is strong self-interest for the health care provider to keep supporting the clinic (as in the project with the residency program), this provides a source of stability and may allow for gradual expansion of goals and vision. Two of the more limited models show how modest goals and a less comprehensive approach may at times lead to a sustainable and successful project.

There has been a growth of school-based health clinics as an alternative way to provide some health care services to underserved children. Many policy experts have pointed out that schools are already a major contact point for all children in this society and especially for poor children. Already in many schools there are programs for free breakfasts and summer food programs in addition to the school lunch program. Some schools are providing after-school care and parenting classes. This is the model of the full-service school approach, as advocated by Dryfoos (1994).

A major question, however, is how sustainable these efforts are without any major state funds (or federal funds through the Maternal and Child Health Block Grant) or some reworking of a state's Medicaid program so that some of those funds might be available to schools. Within Arizona, there are discussions of bills in the legislature that might differentially affect the success of school-based health clinics within Arizona. As part of the tobacco control tax enacted in November 1994, some funds are now being made available to school-based clinics. Some discussion about establishment of funding to follow the model in Florida has occurred. This would offer health insurance with low premiums set on a sliding scale based on eligibility for school lunch. Other discussions are to develop a premium-sharing health insurance plan for the working poor, including those with no children. The state has yet to decide how to incorporate the new federal funds from the Child Health Insurance Program (CHIP). These developments leave many questions unanswered within the state as to how school-based clinics fit within revised arrangements for how health care is provided to poor children. Both at the state and national level, these issues are under discussion.

CHAPTER 6

THE NEED TO PROTECT THE FUTURE

The Impact of Changes in Welfare and Health Policies and Linkages with School Health Issues

What will be decided from the large policy changes underway in both federal welfare and health programs? How will the new State Children's Health Insurance Program (SCHIP) work in different states? How do we as a country view the importance of children, their health care, and special programs for them? All of these questions are important parts of understanding the role of school-based health clinics in the health of children in the 21st century in the United States.

NEW FEDERAL WELFARE PROGRAMS

As was discussed in Chapter 1, the impact of the new federal welfare program is not yet clear. Its goal is to have fewer people on the welfare rolls by moving them into jobs. If the jobs that parents of children formerly on welfare obtain include health insurance for the family, the health care access of these children should improve, even without school-based clinics. If, however, many of these lower-wage jobs do not include health care benefits for family members, parents may earn too much to be Medicaid (or SCHIP) eligible and yet have no other health insurance. For those parents (especially single parents) working a full-time job, taking a child to health care may be difficult. The convenience of being able to obtain care through a school-based health clinic might be important for those parents even if they did have health insurance, especially if the plans included reimbursement for school-based services. One complication is the growth of managed care that is occurring across the United States. For school-based clinics to serve more children in the future, the national association may need to begin to work with large health maintenance organizations (HMOs) on ways to be reimbursed for services. If this could happen, it might also help to provide some recovery of costs through patient fees and to provide a more stable base of funding for some school-based clinics.

For some parents, the incentives to find some health care for their children may increase under the Temporary Assistance for Needy Families (TANF) program (42 §435). Several states are introducing new requirements tying preventive care to welfare benefits. About a third of the states have included an immunization requirement for parents to continue to receive payments. Some states are reducing a family's cash payments if children under age 6 do not receive preventive care, including immunizations. Others are providing a bonus of $20 for each family member over age 8 who obtains health care screenings ("States Experiment," 1997). Although controversy exists within the health care community about whether punitive measures that jeopardize the ability of children to receive food (due to limited money) are a good way to encourage health care requirements, it will be important to follow the impact of these requirements in states over the next few years. In many states, these new requirements began in fiscal year 1997, often only for limited groups initially.

One trend that is occurring is the decline in welfare cases which nationally had reached a record high in March 1994. Since then, caseloads have dropped 18% nationwide, with drops recorded in every state except Hawaii (DeParle, 1997). Most experts attribute the decline in the caseload to the strong economy, not to welfare reform legislation, for most of the decline occurred before the passage of the TANF law in August 1996. Actually, provisions of the TANF law did not begin being implemented until October 1997 or later.

In some ways, the last few years present contradictory trends. The changes in the welfare program are part of what some describe as a new "triumph of meanness" in America. This reflects a political shift to the right that has turned welfare partially back to the states and urged cuts in Head Start while adding funds to the defense budget (Mills, 1997). Other experts have also argued that since the 1980s, the long historical expansion of support systems for child raising has been reversed (Coontz, 1997). Spending on education, child and maternal health, and the infrastructure for future generations has not kept up with increasing needs of the last 20 years. An economist examining issues of children in society has described this as "a mindset . . . extraordinarily careless of children" (Hewlett, 1991, p. 211). Coontz (1997), a historian who has examined myths about the recent American past, has argued that

> the extent to which America has shifted the costs of raising children back onto parents can be seen in the extraordinary retreat from the expansion of public education—a child-centered reform in which the United States once led the world. (p. 143)

In contrast, the passage of SCHIP reflects an expansion of society's role.

SCHIP

The largest expansion of health coverage since the passage of the Medicare and Medicaid Program is the SCHIP effort. Over the 5 years from fiscal year 1998 onward, $24 billion will become available to cover health care for children. Some sources estimate that free or low-cost health care may be provided to up to half of the nation's uninsured children ("Kids' Care," 1997; Kilborn, 1997; "States Hustling," 1997). The program, passed as part of the Balanced Budget Act of 1997 (31 §1321), provides states with much-sought-after flexibility in the ways in which they expand coverage for uninsured children.

The ways in which the new program will work in each state are not yet clear, although there will be options for states to plan very different programs. One option is to use the funds to expand Medicaid eligibility in states. Initial estimates were that at least 11 states would try to implement aspects of the program through Medicaid by increasing eligibility to families earning up to 300% of the poverty level. In Missouri, for example, the state hopes to cover 90,000 additional children who live in families earning up to 300% of the federal poverty level through a fee-for-service Medicaid program ("States Hustling," 1997). More often, states are planning to incorporate more children into managed-care options, often by focusing on families earning up to 200% of the federal poverty level. Another 12 states are planning to implement separate programs, such as those already in place in states such as New York and Minnesota. Some states plan both some Medicaid expansion and some special programs. In many states, coverage to the poorest will be free, with monthly premiums charged as income increases. In the Child Health Plus Plan in New York State, for example, a plan that was covering 114,000 children under age 19 in July 1997, families with incomes between 120 and 160% of the federal poverty level would be charged a maximum premium of $36 a month for a family of four ("New York Tests Limit," 1997).

Some states, such as Florida, will use the funds to expand their Healthy Kids Program started in 1990. This is a school-enrollment-based program that uses school systems as a mechanism to create groups of children large enough to provide a desirable benefit package with relatively low premiums and copayments ("Children's Insurance Programs," 1997). In Florida, boundaries for school districts and counties are the same, making it easier for the state to structure a program that incorporates schools but is administered county by county. In some other states, in which school districts boundaries differ from county lines, it may be easier to distribute funds through public health districts.

Allocation issues across states are important. Under the current Medicaid program, the federal government pays from 50% of the costs in the wealthiest states to 80% in the poorest states. Most states will receive 30% more than they have received in the past through Medicaid, but states must develop specific plans for participation and submit program applications.

Nationally, estimates are that 75% of children eligible for Medicaid because of their family welfare status are currently enrolled ("Kids' Care," 1997). Of nonwelfare children eligible due to past program expansions, 45% are enrolled.

Thus, one major test for the new program will be the actual enrollment rates. Problems with enrollment of eligible children might lead more places to consider school-based programs because schools are in better touch with many eligible children. A school can even plan a case management model of school-based services to help to increase enrollment rates, as was the model in one of the Arizona school-based projects reviewed in Chapter 5.

Health care experts from other countries often are amazed at the complexity of the United States health care system and at the many levels of government involved in new programs. SCHIP will only increase the complexity and variation from one state to another. Though one national program often is viewed by health policy experts as a simpler way to plan a new program, SCHIP provides the opposite situation. The beginning of the 21st century in the United States will see a variety of state programs to provide health insurance to children. States have often been laboratories to discover what types of new programs work or not. It will be important to follow the experiences of different states and their different methods of incorporating SCHIP (and school-based health clinics) into a model of child health care in the United States.

THE FUTURE OF SCHOOL-BASED HEALTH CLINICS

The future of school-based health clinics in the United States is not yet resolved. Major questions are what impact these recently enacted federal changes in welfare policy and child health insurance expansion will have on numbers of children without health insurance. Even if all children had health insurance coverage, however, school-based clinics would still be a useful innovation for many children and their families. Modern families, due to both high rates of divorce and, usually, the need for two incomes, are not likely to have an adult at home full time to cater to the needs of children. Thus, even if costs are not a barrier to receipt of health care, other factors may be, such as the problem of having the time off work to take a child to the health care office and the transportation to take a child to the health care office. For many working parents, being able to have a child receive health care in the school could be a great convenience, and this idea may grow in popularity with parents if the cost of that care can be covered by health insurance (including Medicaid and new special state programs through SCHIP). This is probably most important for parents at the lower end of the economic scale because these are parents who probably have more difficulties with transportation and less flexibility to rearrange their work schedules to obtain health care for their children.

As in the past, when schools were an important resource to help immigrant families accommodate to life in the United States, schools may now be an important resource to help families deal with complex lifestyles and declines in adults' available time to care for children. Schools can provide a support system for busy parents and can make health care both more accessible and affordable, as well as making it culturally acceptable and friendly in the best organized school-based clinics.

The 21st century in the United States may see a return to schools' community involvement and to a role for the school health nurse and school health services that is more integrated with a public health model and with a community wide approach to important services for children. For this to occur, those active in school-based clinics in each state will need to be sure that school-based clinics are included as legitimate providers that can receive reimbursement through the Medicaid program in the state and through whatever mechanisms are used to integrate SCHIP. The growth of managed care in many states, both overall and in the Medicaid program, makes the incorporation of school-based clinics more difficult. If we are to protect the future of children, however, this may be one of the most important policy changes for states to implement. Positive actions by states will be needed to help facilitate the reimbursement of school-based clinics. This will require lobbying by those in favor of school-based clinics and those who advocate for improved child services of all types. Without a more stable financial basis, the innovations will continue to exist in some communities but will not become as widespread a model for receipt of child health care services as could occur with greater interest from state policy makers. Though I and many child policy analysts would agree that children's health programs could benefit from having a structure of a single piece of legislation, such as the Older Americans Act for the elderly, that would address in a consolidated fashion multiple aspects of services, the likelihood of consolidated efforts at the national level is not high in the next few years (Grason & Guyer, 1995). Many health policy experts view SCHIP as a way states will or will not prove to the federal government how worthy they are of the "devolution" trend, in which the federal government cedes responsibility over certain issues to the states ("Kids' Care," 1997). At this juncture, just as state and local governments are very important in overall school policy, they are also very important in the options and programs that are developed to protect the health of children, the group in the population that represents the future of the country.

REFERENCES

Aber, J. L., Bennet, N. G., Conley, D. C., & Li, J. (1997). The effects of poverty on child health and development. *Annual Review of Public Health*, 18, 463-483.

Aday, L. A. (1993). At Risk in America. San Francisco: Jossey-Bass.

Allensworth, D., Wyche, J., & Nicoloson, L. (Eds.). (1995). *Defining a comprehensive school health program: An interim statement*. Washington, DC: National Academy Press.

Angle, J., & Wissman, D. A. (1980). The epidemiology of myopia. *American Journal of Epidemiology*, 11, 220-228.

Arizona Department of Health Services. (1996). *Together we care: School-based, school-linked community services*. Directory. Phoenix, AZ. Bureau of Community and Family Health Services.

Arizona Department of Health Services. (1997). *Together we care: School-based, school-linked community services*. Directory. Phoenix, AZ: Bureau of Community and Family Health Services.

Arnold, L. E., & Jensen, P. S. (1995). Attention-deficit d isorders. In H. I. Kaplan & B. J. Saddock (Eds.), *Comprehensive Book of Psychiatry/VI* (Vol. 2, 6th ed.), Baltimore: Williams & Wilkins.

Balassone, M. L., Bell, M., & Peterfruend, N. (1991). A comparison of users and non-users of a school based health and mental health clinic. *Journal of Adolescent Health*, 12, 240-246.

Ballantyne, R. M. (1997, December 11). Legislature must work to broaden health care for kids. *The Arizona Republic*, p. B6.

Becerra, J. E., Hogue, C. J. R., Atrash, H. K., & Perez, N. (1991). Infant mortality among Hispanics. *Journal of the American Medical Association*, 265, 217-221.

Behrman, R. E. (1996). Overview of pediatrics. In R. E. Behrman, R. M. Kliegman, & A. Arvin (Eds.), *Nelson textbook of pediatrics*. Philadelphia: W. B. Saunders Company.

Beilenson, P. L., Miola, E. S., & Farmer, M. (1995). Politics and practice: Introducing Norplant into a school based health center in Baltimore. *American Journal of Public Health*, 85, 309-311.

Bell, W. (1965). *Aid to Dependent Children*. New York: Columbia University Press.

Bergmann, B. R. (1994). Curing child poverty in the United States. *Papers and Proceedings From the American Economics Association*, 84, 76-80.

Berkowitz, E., & McQuaid, K. (1980). *Creating the welfare state: The political economy of twentieth-century reform*. New York: Praeger.

Borenstein, P. E., Harvilchuck, J D., Rosenthal, B. H., & Santelli, J. S. (1996). Patterns of ICD-9 diagnoses among adolescents using school-based clinics: Diagnostic categories by school level and gender. *Journal of Adolescent Health*, 18, 203-210.

Bradford, B. J., Heald, P. A., Benedum, K. J., & Petrie, S. E. (1996). Immunization status of children on school entry: Area analysis and recommendations. *Clinical Pediatrics*, 25, 237-242.

Bradley, B. J. (1997). The school nurse as health educator. *Journal of School Health*, 67, 3-8.

Brindis, C. (1995). Promising approaches for adolescent reproductive health service delivery. *Western Journal of Medicine*, 163(Suppl.), 50-56.

Brindis, C., Kapphahn, C., McCarter, V., & Wolfe, A. (1995). The impact of health insurance status on adolescents' utilization of school-based clinic services: Implications for health services reform. *Journal of Adolescent Health*, 16, 18-25.

Burnham, J. C. (1982). American medicine's golden age: What happened to it? *Science*, 215, 1474-1479.

Butler, J., Rosenbaum, S., & Palfrey, J. S. (1987). Ensuring access to health care for children with disabilities. *New England Journal of Medicine*, 317, 162-165.

Butterfoss, F. D., Goodman, R. M., & Wandersman, A. (1993). A community coalition for prevention and health promotion. *Health Education Research*, 8, 315-330.

Cassil, A. (1997, November 17). 86 percent of uninsured kids in NM eligible but not enrolled in Medicaid. *American Medical News*, p. 4.

Centers for Disease Control and Prevention. (1996). Guidelines for school health programs to promote lifelong healthy eating. *Morbidity and Mortality Weekly Report*, 45 (RR-9), 1-41.

Centers for Disease Control and Prevention. (1994). Guidelines for school health programs to prevent tobacco use and addiction. *Morbidity and Mortality Weekly Report*, 43 (RR-2), 1-18.

Center for the Future of Children. (1992). Recommendations and analysis. *Future of Children*, 2(2), 6-25.

Chafel, J. A. (1993). Child poverty: Overview and outlook. In J. A. Chafel (Ed.), *Child poverty and public policy*. Washington, DC: Urban Institute Press.

Children's insurance programs gain new popularity. (1997, April). *State Initiatives in Health Care Reform*, 13(No. 23), 4-7, 12.

Coiro, M. J., Zill, N., & Bloom, B. (1994). Health of our nation's children. (Vital and Health Statistics, Series 10, No. 191). Hyattsville, MD: National Center for Health Statistics.

Collins, J. G., & LeClere, F. B. (1996). Health and selected socioeconomic characteristics of the family, United States, 1988-90. (Vital and Health Statistics, Series 10, No. 195). Hyattsville, MD: National Center for Health Statistics.

Collins, J. W., & David, R. J. (1990). The differential effects of traditional risk factors in infant birth weights among blacks and whites in Chicago. *American Journal of Public Health*, 80, 679-681.

Collins, J. L., Small, M. L., Kahn, L., Pateman, Collins, B., Gold, R. S., & Kolbe, L. (1995). School health education. *Journal of School Health*, 65, 302-311.

Coontz, S. (1997). *The Way We really Are: Coming To Terms with America's Changing Families*. New York: Basic Books.

Costello, E. (1989). Child psychiatric disorders and their correlates: A primary care pediatric sample. *Journal of the American Academy of Child and Adolescent Psychiatry*, 28, 851-855.

Cortese, P. A. (1993). Accomplishments in comprehensive school health education. *Journal of School Health*, 63, 21-23.

Davis, T., & Allensworth, D. D. (1994). Program management: A necessary component for the comprehensive school health program. *Journal of School Health*, 64, 400-404.

DeParle, J. (1997, February 23). A sharp decrease in welfare cases is gathering speed. *New York Times*, p. 1, 12.

Donabedian, A. (1980). *Exploration in quality assessment and monitoring: Vol. 1. The definition of quality and approaches to its assessments*. Ann Arbor, MI: Health Administration Press.

Dryfoos, J. G. (1994). *Full-service schools: A revolution in health and social services for children, youth and families*. San Francisco: Jossey-Bass.

Duncan, G. J., & Rodgers, W. (1988). Has children's poverty become more consistent? *American Sociological Review*, 56, 538-550.

Exploring national issues and priorities. (1996). *Journal of School Nursing*, 12, 23-36.

Fingerhut, L., & Kleinman, J. (1989). *Trends and current status in childhood mortality, U.S., 1900-1985*. (Vital and Health Statistics, Series 2, No. 26). Hyattsville, MD: National Center for Health Statistics.

Fischer, M., Juszczark, L., Friedman, S. B., Schneider, M., & Chapar, G. (1992). School based adolescent health care: A review of a clinical service. *American Journal of Diseases of the Child*, 146, 615-621.

Fix, M., & Zimmerman, W. (1993). *Educating Immigrant Children*. Washington, DC: Urban Institute Press.

Flaherty, L. T., Weist, M. D., & Warner, B. S. (1996). School-based mental health services in the United States: History, current models and needs. *Community Mental Health Journal*, 32, 341-352.

Francis, E., Esielionis, H., Persis, J., Treolar, D. M., & Yarandi, H. (1996). Who dispenses pharmacueticals to children at school? *Journal of School Health*, 66, 355-358.

Fryer, G. E., & Igoe, J. B. (1996). Functions of school nurses and health assistants in U.S. school health programs. *Journal of School Health*, 66, 55-63.

Galavotti, C., & Lovick, S. R. (1989). School based clinic use and other factors affecting adolescent contraceptive behavior. *Journal of Adolescent Health* Care, 10, 506-512.

Gergen, P. J., Mullally, D. I., & Evans, R. (1988). National survey of prevalence of asthma among children in the United States. *Pediatrics*, 81, 1-7.

Gotsch-Thompson, S. (1988). Ideology and welfare reform under the Reagan administration. In D. Tomaskovic-Devey, (Ed.), *Poverty and Social Welfare in the United States*. Boulder, CO: Westview Press.

Grason, H., & Guyer, B. (1995). Rethinking the organization of children's programs: Lessons from the elderly. *The Milbank Quarterly*, 73, 565-597.

Green, M., & Solnit, A. J. (1964). Reactions to the threatened loss of a child: A vulnerable child syndrome. *Pediatrics*, 34, 58-66.

Guyer, B., & Ellers, B. (1990). Childhood injuries in the U.S. *American Journal of Diseases of Children*, 144, 659-652.

Hacker, K. (1996). Integrating school-based health centers into managed care in Massachusetts. *Journal of School Health*, 66, 317-321.

Hacker, K., Fried, L. E., Bablouzian, L., & Roeber, J. (1994). A nationwide survey of school health services delivery in urban schools. *Journal of School Health*, 64, 279-283.

Hadley, J. (1982). More medical care! Better health? In J. Hadley (Ed.), *Economic Analysis of Mortality Rates*. Washington, DC: The Urban Institute.

Haggerty, R. J. (1983). Epidemiology of childhood disease. In D. Mechanic (Ed.), *Handbook of Health, Health Care and the Health Professions*. (pp. 101-119). New York: Free Press.

Handler, J. F. (1995). *The Poverty of Welfare Reform*. New Haven, CT: Yale University Press.

Handler, J. F., & Hasenfeld, Y. (1991). *The Moral Construction of Poverty: American Welfare Reform*. Newbury Park, CA: Sage.

Harrison, B. A., Faircloth, J. W., & Yaryan, L. (1995). The impact of legislation on the role of the school nurse. *Nursing Outlook*, 43, 57-61.

Harold, R. D., & Harold, N. B. (1993). School-based clinics: A response to the physical and mental health needs of adolescents. *Health and Social Work*, 18, 65-74.

Hawkins, J., Hayes, E. R., & Corliss, P. (1994). School nursing in America - 1902-1994: A Return to public health nursing. Public Health Nursing, 11, 416-425.

Hewlett, S. (1991). *When the Bough Breaks*. New York: Basic Books.

Hofferth, S. (1993). The 101st Congress: An emerging agenda for children in poverty. In J. A. Chafel (Ed.), *Child Poverty and Public Policy*. Washington, DC: Urban Institute Press.

Igoe, J. B. (1994). School nursing. *Nursing Clinics of North America*, 29, 443-458.

Institute of Medicine. (1989). *Research on Children and Adolescents with Mental, Behavioral and Developmental Disorders: Mobilizing a National Initiative*. Washington, DC: National Academy Press.

Irwin, C. E., & Millstein, S. G. (1986). Biopsychosocial correlates of risk-taking behavior in adolescence. *Journal of Adolescent Health Care*, 7, 82s-92s.

Johnston, L. D., Bachman, J. G., & O'Malley, P. M. (1984). *Use of Licit and Illicit Drugs by America's High School Students*. (DHHS Publication No. 85-1394). Rockville, MD: National Institute of Drug Abuse.

Joining Hands: News From the National Assembly on School-Based Health Care. (1995). (Vol. 1, No. 1). McLean, VA: National Assembly on School-Based Health Care.

Kahn, L., Collins, J. L., Pateman, B. C., Small, M. L., Ross, J. G., & Kolbe, L. J. (1995). The School Health Policies and Programs Study (SHPPS): Rationale for a nationwide status report on school health programs. *Journal of School Health*, 65, 291-294.

Kaplan, D. W. (1995). School-based health centers: Primary care in high school. *Pediatric Annals*, 24, 192-200.

Keyl, P., Hurtado, M. P., Barber, M. M., & Borton, J. (1996). School-based health centers: Students' access, knowledge and use of services. *Archives of Pediatric and Adolescent Medicine*, 150, 175-180.

Kids care tests whether states can handle big-time responsibility. (1997, November 10). *American Hospital Association News*, 33, 3.

Kilborn, P. T. (1997, September 21). States to provide health insurance to more children. *The New York Times*, pp. 1, 22.

King, C. R. (1993). *Children's Health in America.* New York: Maxwell Macmillan International.

Kirby, D. (1992). *Research Methods For Assessing and Evaluating School-Based Clinics.* Washington, DC: Center for Population Options.

Kitzman, H., Olds, D. L., Henderson, C. R., Hanks, C., Cole, R., Tatelbaun, R., McConnochie, K. M., Sidora, K., Luckey, D. W., Shaver, D., Engelhardt, K., James, D., & Barnard, K. (1997). Effect of prenatal and infancy home visitation on pregnancy, outcomes, childhood injuries, and repeated childbearing. *Journal of the American Medical Association*, 278, 644-652.

Klein, J. D., & Cox, E. M. (1995). School-based health clinics in the mid 1990s. *Current Opinion in Pediatrics*, 7, 353-359.

Kogan, M. D., Alexander, G. R., Teitelbaum, M. A., Jack, B. W., Kotelchuck, M., & Pappas, G. (1995). The effect of gaps in health insurance on continuity of a regular source of care among preschool-aged children in the United States. *Journal of the American Medical Association*, 274, 1430-1435.

Kolbe, L. D. (1993). Developing a plan of action to institutionalize school health education programs in the United States. *Journal of School Health*, 63, 12-13.

Krieger, N., Rowley, D., Herman, A. A., Avery, B., & Phillips, M. T. (1993). Racism, sexism, and social class: Implications for studies of health, disease and well-being. *American Journal of Preventive Medicine*, 9(Suppl. 6), 82-122.

Kronenfeld, J. J., & Whicker, M. L. (1984). *US National Health Policy: An Analysis of the Federal Role.* New York: Praeger.

Kronenfeld, J. J. (1998). *The Changing Federal Role in U.S. Health Care Policy.* Westport, CT: Praeger Publishers.

Kronenfeld, J. J. (1996). *Flinn Final Report: Evaluation of School Health Projects and Extended Evaluations As New Projects Were Added.* Flinn Foundation: Phoenix, AZ.

Lavin, A. T. (1993). Comprehensive school health education: barriers and opportunities. *Journal of School Health*, 63, 24-27.

Lear, J. G., Montgomery, L. L., Schlitt, J. J., & Rickett, K. D. (1996). Key issues affecting school-based health centers and Medicaid. *Journal of School Health*, 66, 83-88.

Lear, J. G., Gleicher, H. B., St. Germaine, A., & Porter, P. J. (1991). Reorganizing health care for adolescents: The experience of the school-based adolescent health care program. *Journal of Adolescent Health*, 12, 450-458.

Leff, M. (1983). Consensus for reform: The mothers'-pension movement in the Progressive Era. *Social Service Review*, 47, 397-417.

Levine, M. D. (1982). The high-prevalence-low-severity developmental disorders of school children. *Advances in Pediatrics*, 29, 529-544.

Levine, M. D., & Satz, P. (1984). *Middle Childhood: Development and Dysfunction.* Baltimore: University Park Press.

Levy, J. C. (1980). Vulnerable children: Parents' perceptions and the use of medical care. *Pediatrics*, 65, 956-963.

Lewit, E. M. (1992). Teenage childbearing. In *The Future of Children*, 2(2), 186-191.

Lipper, E. G., Farr, M., Marchese, C., Palfrey, J., & Darby, B. J. (1997). Partnerships in school care. *American Journal of School Health, 87, 291-293.*

Lytle, L. E., Johnson, C. C., Bachman, K., Wambsgans, K., Perry, C. L., Stone, E. J., & Budman, S. (1994). Successful recruitment strategies for school-based health promotion: Experiences from CATCH. *Journal of School Health*, 64, 405-409.

Markides, K. S., & Coreil, J. (1986). The health of Hispanics in the southwestern United States. *Public Health Reports*, 101, 253-265.

Marks, E. L., & Marzke, C. H. (1993). *Health Caring: A Process Evaluation of the Robert Wood Johnson Foundation's School-Based Adolescent Health Care Program.* Princeton, NJ: Mathtech, Inc.

Massey, J. T. (1989). Design and Estimation for the National Health Interview Survey, 1985-1994. (Vital and Health Statistics, Series 10, No. 173). Hyattsville, MD: National Center for Health Statistics.

Maurer, H. M. (1993). Growing neglect of American children. *American Journal of Diseases of the Child*, 147, 259.

Maynard, R. A., (Ed.). (1997). Kids Having Kids. New York: The Urban Institute.

McCord, M., Klein, J. D., Foy, J. M., & Fothergill, K. (1993). School-based clinic use and school performance. *Journal of Adolescent Health*, 14, 91-98.

McCormack, M. C., & Brooks-Gunn, J. (1989). The health of children and adolescents. In H. E. Freeman & S. Levine, (Eds.), *Handbook of Medical Sociology* (4th ed.). Englewood Cliffs, NJ: Prentice-Hall.

McCormick, M. C., Brooks-Gunn, J., Workman-Daniels, K., & Peckham, G. (1993). Maternal rating of child health at school age: Does the vulnerable child syndrome persist? *Pediatrics*, 92, 380-388.

McCormick, M. C. (1987). Implications of recent changes in infant mortality. In L. H. Aiken, & D. Mechanic, (Eds.), *Applications of Social Science to Clinical Medicine and Health Policy*, (pp. 282-306). New Brunswick, NJ: Rutgers University Press.

McGinnis, J. M. (1993). The year 2000 initiative: Implications for comprehensive school health education. *Preventive Medicine*, 22, 493-498.

Michigan Model for Comprehensive School Health Education - Implementation Plan for the Year 1991. (1991). East Lansing, MI: State of Michigan.

Miller, A. C., Fine, A., & Adams-Taylor, S. (1989). *Monitoring Children's Health Care: Key Indicators (2nd ed.).* Washington, DC: American Public Health Association.

Mills, N. (1997). *The Triumph of Meanness: America's War Against Its Better Self.* Boston: Houghton Mifflin.

Moffitt, T. E. (1997). Helping poor mothers and children. *Journal of the American Medical Association*, 278, 680-681.

Murray, C. (1984). *Losing Ground: American Social Policy, 1950-1980.* New York: Basic.

National Association of State School Nurse Consultants. (1996). Delegation of school health services to unlicenced personnel: A position paper. *Journal of School Health*, 66, 72-74.

National Commission on Children. (1991). *Beyond Rhetoric: A New American Agenda for Children and Families.* Washington, DC: National Commission on Children.

Neumark-Sztainer, D. (1996). School-based programs for preventing eating disturbances. *Journal of School Health*, 66, 64-71.

Newacheck, P., Jameson, W. J., & Halfon, N. (1994). Health status and income: The impact of poverty on child health. *Journal of School Health*, 64, 229-233.

Newacheck, P., & Starfield, B. (1988). Morbidity and use of ambulatory care services among poor and non-poor children. *American Journal of Public Health*, 78, 927-933.

Newacheck, P., & Stoddard, J. (1994). Prevalence and impact of multiple childhood chronic illnesses. *The Journal of Pediatrics*, 124, 40-48.

Newacheck, P. W., & Taylor, W. R. (1992). Childhood chronic illness: Prevalence, severity and impact. *American Journal of School Health*, 82, 364-371.

New York tests limits of benefit package and affordability as it aims to double size of children's insurance plan. (1997, July) *State Health Watch*, 4(No. 7). pp. 2, 8.

Nickens, H. W. (1995). The role of race/ethnicity and social class in minority health status. *Health Services Research*, 30 (No. 1, Part II), 151-161.

Novella, A. C., Wise, P. H., & Kleinman, D. V. (1991). Hispanic health: Time for data, time for action. *New England Journal of Medicine*, 265, 254-255.

The number of Americans. (1995, March-April). *State Initiatives in Health Care Reform*, 11, 1-3.

Number of school-based health centers increasing. (1997, April). *The Nation's Health* p. 11.

Oberg, C. N., Bryant, N. A., & Bach, M. L. (1994). *America's Children: Triumph or Tragedy*. Washington, DC: American Public Health Association.

Olds, D. L., Eckenrode, J., Henderson, C. R., Kitzman, H., Powers, J., Cole, R., Sidora, K., Morris, P., Pettit, L. M., & Luckey, D. (1997). Long-term effects of home visitation on maternal life course and child abuse and neglect. *Journal of the American Medical Association*, 278, 637-643.

Orshansky, M. (1965). Counting the poor: another look at the poverty profile. *Social Security Bulletin*, 28, 3-29.

Pappas, G., Queen, S., Hadden, W., & Fisher, G. (1993). The increasing disparity in mortality between socioeconomic groups in the United States, 1960 and 1986. *New England Journal of Medicine*, 329, 103-109.

Passarelli, C. (1994). School nursing: Trends for the future. *Journal of School Health*, 64, 141-149.

Patrick, D., & Elinson, J. (1979). Methods of sociomedical research. In N. Freeman, H. E. Levine, & L. G. Reeder (Eds.), *Handbook of Medical Sociology* (3rd ed.), (pp. 483-500). Englewood Cliffs, NJ: Prentice-Hall.

Patterson, J. T. (1981). *America's Struggle Against Poverty, 1900-1980*. Cambridge, MA: Harvard University Press.

Perrin, J., Guyer, B., & Lawrence, J. M. (1992). Health care services for children and adolescents. *The Future of Children*, 2(2), 59-77.

Pickett, G., & Hanlon, J. (1990). *Public Health: Administration and Practice*. St. Louis, MO: Times Mirror/Mosby College Publishing.

Piven, F. F., & Cloward, R. A. (1971). *Regulating The Poor: The Functions of Public Welfare*. New York: Academic Press.

Pless, I., & Roghman, K. (1971). Childhood illness and its consequences: Observations based on three epidemiological surveys. *The Journal of Pediatrics*, 79, 351-359.

Pollitt, P. (1994). The first school nurse. *Journal of School Nursing*, 10, 34-36.

Proctor, S., Lordi, S., & Zeiger, D. (1993). *School Nursing Practice: Roles and Standards*. Scarborough, ME: National Association of School nurses.

Quick updates - making the grade in school health. (1997). *Journal of the American Medical Association*, 277, 1270.

Racine, A. D., Joyce, T. J., & Grossman, M. (1992). Effectiveness of health care services for pregnant women and infants. *The Future of Children*, 2(2), 40-57.

Rajsky-Steed, N. (1996). The nurse practitioner in the school setting. *Advanced Practice Nursing*, 31, 507-518.

Rickert, V. I., Davis, S. O., & Ryan, S. (1997). Rural school-based clinics: Are adolescents willing to use them and what services do they want? *Journal of School Health*, 67,

144-148.

Roberts, J. (1973). Examination and health history findings among children and youth 6-17 years. (Vital and Health Statistics, Series 11, No. 129). Hyattsville, MD: National Center for Health Statistics.

Roberts, L. (1922). The nutrition and care of children in a mountain county of Kentucky. *Children's Bureau Publication* (No. 10). Washington, DC: U. S. Department of Health, Education, Welfare, and Rehabilitation Services.

Salmon, M. E. (1994). School health nursing in the era of health care reform: What is the outlook? *Journal of School Health*, 64, 137-140.

Sanders, J. M. (1988). A test of the new structural critique of the welfare state. In D. Tomaskovic-Devey (Ed.), *Poverty and Social Welfare in the United States*, (pp. 130-161). Boulder, CO: Westview Press.

Santelli, J., Kouzis, A., & Newcomer, S. (1996). School-based health centers and adolescent use of primary care and hospital care. *Journal of Adolescent Health*, 19, 267-275.

Scarbrough, W. H. (1993). Who are the poor: A demographic perspective. In J. A. Chafel (Ed.), *Child Poverty and Public Policy*. Washington, DC: Urban Institute Press.

Schlitt, J. J., Rickett, K., Montgomery, L. L., & Lear, J. G. (1995). State initiatives to support school-based health centers: A national survey. *Journal of Adolescent Health*, 17, 68-76.

Schoendorf, K. D., Hogue, C. J. R., Kleinman, J. C., & Rowley, D. (1992). Mortality among infants of black as compared with white college-educated parents. *New England Journal of Medicine*, 326, 1522-1526.

School-Based Health Centers Can Expand Access for Children. (1994, December). Report to the Chairman, Committee on Government Operations, House of Representatives. Washington, DC: General Accounting Office, HEHS 95093.

School-based centers search for funding: Eye managed care organizations as partners. (1994, September-October). *State Initiatives in Health Care Reform*, 10(No. 14), pp. 7-9.

Sherman, A. (1994). *Wasting's America's Future: The Chidlren's Defense Fund Report on the Costs of Child Poverty*. Boston: Beacon Press.

Skocpol, T. (1992). *Protecting Soldiers and Mothers: The Political Origins of Social Policy in the United States*. Cambridge, MA: Harvard University Press.

Sliepcevich, E. (1982). *Health Education: A Conceptual Approach to Curriculum Design*. St. Paul, MN: 3M Education Press.

Small, M., Leavy, M., Smith, L., Allensworth, D. D., Farhquhar, B. K., Kann, L., & Pateman, B. C. (1995). School health services. *Journal of School Health*, 65, 319-325.

Society for Adolescent Medicine. (1992). Access to health care for adolescents: A position paper of the Society for Adolescent Medicine. *Journal of Adolescent Health*, 13, 162-170.

Sowell, T. (1983). *The Economics and Politics of Race: An Economic Perspective*. New York: William Morrow.

States experiment with using welfare as leverage to get preventive care for children. (1997, July). *State Health Watch*, 4, pp. 3, 11.

States hustling to get their share of $24 billion for kids' coverage. (1997, November 10). *American Hospital Association News*, 33, 5-6.

Status report on the childhood immunization initiative. (1997). *Morbidity and Mortality Weekly Report*, 46, 57-664.

Starfield, B. (1985). *The Effectiveness of Medical Care Validating Clinical Wisdom.* Baltimore, MD: Johns Hopkins University Press.

Starfield, B. (1991). Childhood morbidity: Comparisons, clusters, and trends. *Pediatrics,* 88, 519-526.

Starfield, B., Bergner, M., Ensminger, M., Riley, A., Ryan, S., Green, B., McGauhey, P., Skinner, A., & Kim, S. (1993). Adolescent health status measurement: Development of the child health and illness profile. *Pediatrics,* 91, 430-435.

Starfield, B., Forrest, C. B., Ryan, S., Riley, A., Ensminger, M. E., & Green, B. F. (1996). Health status of well versus ill adolescents. *Archives of Pediatric and Adolescent Medicine,* 1, 1249-1256.

Starfield, B., Riley, A., Green, B., Ensminger, M., Ryan, S., Kelleher, K., Kim-Harris, S., & Vogel, K. (1995). The adolescent child health and illness profile. *Medical Care,* 33, 553-566.

The state of school nursing today. (1995). *Journal of School Health,* 65, 371-389.

Terwilliger, S. H. (1994). Early access to health care services through a rural school-based health center. *Journal of School Health,* 64, 284-289.

Tokarski, C. (1995). Healthier times at Ridgemont High. *Hospitals and Health Networks,* 69, 36-38.

Tomaskovic-Devey, D. (1988). *Poverty and Social Welfare in the United States.* Boulder, CO: Westview Press.

U.S. Congress, Office of Technology Assessment. (1991). *Adolescent Health, Volume 1: Summary and Policy Options.* (OTA-H-468). Washington, DC: U.S. Government Printing Office.

U.S. Department of Health and Human Services. (1991). *Healthy People 2000: National Health Promotion and Disease Prevention Objectives.* Washington, DC: Public Health Service.

Urbinati, D., Steele, P., Harter, B. J. E., & Harrell, D. (1996). The evolution of the school nurse practitioner: Past, present and future. *Journal of School Nursing,* 12, 6-9.

Walter, H. J., Vaughan, R. D., Armstrong, B., Krakoff, R. Y., Tiezzi, L., & McCarthy, J. F. (1996). Characteristics of user and nonusers of school clinics in inner city junior high schools. *Journal of Adolescent Health,* 18, 344-348.

Watts, J. (1997). The end of work and the end of welfare: Review of the Personal Responsibility and Work Opportunity Reconciliation Act of 1996. *Contemporary Sociology,* 26, 409-412.

Weist, M. D., Paskewitz, D. A., Warner, B. S., & Flaherty, L. T. (1996). Treatment outcome of school-based mental health services for urban teenagers. *Community Mental Health Journal,* 32, 149-157.

Wenzel, M. (1996). A school-based clinic for elmentary schools in Arizona. *Journal of School Health,* 66, 125-127.

While, A. E., & Barriball, K. L. (1993). School nursing: History, present practice, and possibilities reviewed. *Journal of Advanced Nursing,* 18, 1202-1211.

Williams, J. K., & McCarthy, A. M. (1995). School nurses' experience with children with chronic conditions. *Journal of School Health,* 65, 234-236.

Yates, S. (1994a, February). Integration with new models of health service delivery. *Journal of School Nursing,* 10(No. 1), 10-14.

Yates, S. (1994b, April). School health delivery programs throughout the United States. *Journal of School Nursing,* 10(No. 2), 31-36.

Yawn, B., Lydick, E. G., Epstein, R., & Jacobsen, S. J. (1996). Is health vision screening effective? *Journal of School Health*, 66, 171-175.

Zill, N., & Schoenborn, C. A. (1990). Developmental, learning and emotional problems: Health of our nation's children, United States, 1988. (Advance Data From Vital and Health Statistics, No. 190). Hyattsville, MD: National Center for Health Statistics.

Zimmerman, D. J., & Reif, C. J. (1995). School-based health centers and managed care health plans: Partners in primary care. *Journal of Public Health Management Practice*, 1(1), 33-39.

Index

ABOUT THE AUTHOR

Jennie Jacobs Kronenfeld is a Professor in the School of Health Administration and Policy, College of Business, Arizona State University at Tempe. She holds a doctorate (1976) and a master's (1973) in sociology from Brown University and a BA (1971) in sociology and history at the University of North Carolina, Chapel Hill. Before coming to Arizona, she held faculty positions at the University of Alabama in Birmingham and the University of South Carolina. She has published over 80 articles in public health, medicine, and sociology. She has authored or coauthored 12 books, one in 1981 on the social and economic aspects of coronary artery bypass surgery; one in 1984 on the federal role in health policy; one in 1986 on the impact of technology on sex roles and social change; one in 1990 on social policies and privatization issues in the care of the young, the sick, the imprisoned, and the elderly; one in 1993 on controversial issues in health policy, and several relating to career strategies in academe (tenure, ethical concerns, and the job search). Several recent edited books are part of the research annual series of *Research in the Sociology of Health Care*, for which she has served as the editor or co-editor since 1993. She has held numerous national offices in various professional sociological and health association. She currently teaches courses on health care policy; social, economic, and political factors in health care; and methodological issues in health care research.